A guide to prevention in dentistry

including

Prevention

and

The scientific basis of oral health education

Prevention

Professor Elizabeth Kay of Dental Health Services Research,
University of Manchester Dental Hospital and School,
Higher Cambridge Street, Manchester M15 6FH

2004
Published by the British Dental Association
64 Wimpole Street, London, W1G 8YS

ISBN 0 904588 85 8 (Softback)
ISBN 0 904588 86 6 (Hardback)

Cover photograph courtesy of
Irfan Ahmad (iahmadbds@aol.com)

Printed and bound by
Dennis Barber Limited, Lowestoft, Suffolk

Contents

Preface

In 1997, Professor David Locker, of the University of Toronto, and I published a review of the evidence underpinning oral health promotion. That review was widely misquoted as saying that 'oral health promotion does not work'. In actual fact, what the review demonstrated was that the evidence base for oral health promotion was, in general, weak and that there were very few robust trials available to support our oral health promotion and disease prevention efforts. However, what the review also revealed was that the strongest evidence suggested that fluoride was a crucial part of the preventive practitioner armamentarium. Perhaps even more importantly and, it must be said, somewhat unexpectedly, the findings of the review showed that chairside, one-to-one advice from a dental health professional was a useful and powerful preventive tool.

This new book, therefore, aims to assist the preventive-oriented dental professional by providing them with the latest thinking on various aspects of prevention. It also aims to advise them of the strength of the evidence underpinning the things they do. Most importantly, in the preparation of the text, I was determined that the information contained within the book should not be simply the 'received wisdom' of the oral health promotion 'experts' but instead should provide an authoritative and evidence-based review of the current state-of-the-art in various aspects of chairside prevention. Most importantly, I wanted the book to be written by people who were actually researching, and working, on a day to day basis, with the people and agents under review. Thus, this book is authored by an eclectic mix of researchers, who are drawn from different parts of the world. At times, this pursuit of the right academic to author each chapter has led to variation in style and emphasis between the different parts of the book. However, one constant which does run through it, is assessment of the strength of the evidence-base underpinning each of the authors' suggestions and recommendations.

Dentistry currently stands at a crossroads, but, with the advent of the new contract, with the loss of fee-for-item-of-service remuneration, and with the advent of a mandatory oral health assessment, it is inconceivable that preventive dentistry will not become a much more important part of a general dental practitioner's day to day business. Furthermore, the burgeoning of the size of professions complementary to dentistry and the rapid increase in their responsibilities will mean that clear and consistent preventive messages are of ever greater importance for dental teams. This book will, we hope, provide teams with clear guidance, but, crucially, the preventive messages this book advises are underpinned by research evidence.

Elizabeth Kay

May 2004

Acknowledgements

Firstly, I must thank the authors of the papers in this book, who worked so diligently. They willingly redrafted their work in order for us to try to achieve consistency between the chapters, and to ensure that they classified the evidence they were using. I am proud of the result and very much hope that they are too.

Secondly, I must thank Miss Pam Brown. Without her help and patient coordination of this worldwide group of dental academics (by their own admission, not the easiest people to organise!) these papers would never have been written, or assembled into a book. Her perseverance and forbearance are extraordinary and I am deeply grateful to her for her work on this book, and for many other things.

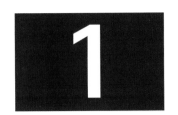

IN BRIEF

- Prevention is a fundamental element of clinical practice. This is the first in a series of papers which will review and update the evidence base for preventive action in general dental practice.
- One important, but underdeveloped area of prevention is smoking cessation. Smoking and tobacco use adversely affects oral health in a variety of ways. The dental profession and their teams have a potentially important role to play in helping smokers to quit.
- This paper aims to review the practical steps that the dental team can implement in smoking cessation activities within the clinical dental setting.

Prevention. Part 1: Smoking cessation advice within the general dental practice

R. G. Watt[1] and B. Daly[2]; Series Editor E. J. Kay[3]

Smoking remains the largest single preventable cause of death and disability in the UK and costs the NHS £1.7 billion each year.[1] More than 120,000 people die prematurely due to smoking related diseases. Worldwide smoking is the single most important public health problem. The detrimental effects of smoking and tobacco use on oral health are well recognised. Oral cancers and pre-cancers, periodontal diseases and poor wound healing are the most significant and serious effects of smoking on the mouth.[2,3] In addition, staining of the teeth, soft tissue changes and halitosis are aesthetic and social impacts of smoking directly related to oral health.

[1]*Reader, Department of Epidemiology and Public Health, Royal Free and University College London Medical School, University College London, 1-19 Torrington Place, London WC1E 6BT; [2]Lecturer, Department of Dental Public Health, The Guy's, Kings and St. Thomas' Schools of Medicine, Dentistry and Biomedical Sciences. GKT Dental Institute, Caldecot Road, London SE5 9RW
[3]Professor of Dental Health Services Research, University of Manchester Dental Hospital and School, Higher Cambridge Street, Manchester M15 6FH
*Correspondence to: R G Watt
E-mail: r.watt@ucl.ac.uk

Recently published evidence-based guidelines on smoking cessation have highlighted the important role that health professionals can play in helping smokers to stop successfully.[4] Systematic reviews of many randomised controlled trials have shown the effectiveness of smoking cessation advice provided by general medical practitioners. On the recognised hierarchy of evidence, these would be classified as Type 1 evidence. Relatively few well designed studies have been undertaken to assess the effectiveness of dental professionals in smoking cessation activities although the success rates achieved are comparable with studies in other primary care settings.[5,6] Indeed factors such as access to smokers, level of training, experience and commitment are more important in determining success than professional discipline.[7]

Although many dentists express positive attitudes to becoming actively involved in smoking cessation activities with their patients, few routinely assist smokers to stop.[8,9] This paper aims to outline ways in which dental practitioners and their teams can support smokers to effectively quit. Very limited time is required when assistance and support is provided in a standardised way to those smokers interested and willing to stop. Involvement in smoking cessation provides an opportunity for dentists to become engaged in an interesting, relevant and important area of prevention.

WHO SMOKES ANYMORE?

In the UK around 28% of the adult population smoke, that is over 13 million smokers.[10]

Although the overall rate of smoking has declined steadily since the 1940s, smoking is now increasingly restricted to the more disadvantaged sections of society. For example, in 1996, 12% of men in professional occupations smoked compared with 40% of men in unskilled manual jobs.[11] Although dental attendance is inversely related to deprivation, many smokers will be seen by general dental practitioners.

Across many parts of the developed world concern has been expressed about the continuing problem of teenage smokers, especially amongst young women. The vast majority of adult smokers start during their adolescence. Once started, although many smokers report a desire to give up, they will become addicted to nicotine and will spend years struggling to break the habit.

TIME FOR ACTION

Based upon a systematic review of the scientific evidence, a smoking cessation protocol has been published and updated to encourage health professionals, including dentists to become more actively involved in smoking prevention.[4,11] The 4 A's model is a straightforward and quick means of identifying smokers who want to stop and how best to help them achieve their goal (Fig. 1).

Advice and support provided in a clinical setting will be most effective with patients who are interested and keen to make a quit attempt. Pressurising 'contented' smokers will most often achieve very little. It is essential to tailor advice and support to smokers who are ready and willing to change their behaviour. The use of appro-

Table 1 Questioning techniques and styles

- Use both closed and open questions, as appropriate, depending on what information you require
- Give patients time to answer your questions – don't rush them!
- Encourage patients to speak openly and honestly
- Take care not to be seen as nagging or judgemental – this achieves nothing
- Sum up any information given to you to check you have understood what has been said

priate questioning techniques is therefore very important (Table 1).

The different steps in the 4 A's model will now be outlined.

Ask

All patients should have their smoking status checked at the start of each course of treatment. A simple and quick system should be devised to record smoking details in the patient's clinical notes. This information should be kept up to date as possible. The following questions can be used within a standard medical history to assess whether the patient smokes, their level of nicotine addiction and their motivation to stop.

Are you a smoker?
How many cigarettes do you smoke each day?
How soon after waking up in the morning do you have your first cigarette?
Have you ever tried to stop smoking?
Are you interested in stopping now?

Patients who report smoking more than 20 cigarettes per day and who have their first cigarette within 30 minutes of waking up in the morning are likely to be heavily dependent upon nicotine and will require more specialised and intensive support. These individuals are best referred to the local specialist services for help.

Advise

All smokers and those using other forms of tobacco should be advised of the value of stopping. The advice should be clear, firm and personally relevant. Although most people are aware of the harmful effects of smoking in relation to lung cancer and heart disease, fewer people know about the detrimental effects of smoking on their oral health.[12] This provides a unique opportunity for dentists and members of the team to highlight the dangers of smoking in what could be considered an appropriate setting, the dental surgery. Scarring patients with frightening images of diseased organs may not be effective for many people. Instead a range of reasons for stopping smoking could be highlighted, some directly related to oral health, others more general (Table 2). Consider what is likely to be most significant and relevant to the patient. For example, stained teeth, halitosis and soft tissue changes in the mouth may be especially pertinent to young people. The early effects of tobacco use on the mouth are visible and reversible and may be a useful means of motivating smokers on the benefits of stopping. All smokers however will have their own good reasons for stopping.

Assist

If during the first two stages a smoker expresses a desire to quit, help and support should be offered. For those smokers not ready or willing to give up at this point, it is best raising the issue

ASK
All patients should have their smoking status checked

⇩

ADVISE
All smokers should be advised on the value of quitting

⇩

ASSIST
For those smokers who want to stop, appropriate support should be offered

⇩

ARRANGE
Monitoring, follow up and referral should be arranged as appropriate

Fig. 1 The four A's approach to smoking cessation

again at a later stage to check if they have changed their opinions. Putting pressure or nagging smokers who are not ready to quit can be counterproductive and a waste of your and their time.

Assistance for those wishing to quit should focus on the following points:

- Negotiate a quit date – smokers need time to prepare
- Review past experiences of quitting – identify what helped and hindered progress in the past
- Identify any potential problems ahead and plan how these can be dealt with
- Stress the importance of enlisting the support of friends, family and colleagues – their assistance is essential
- Explore the value of using nicotine replacement therapy and Bupropion (Zyban) (see below for further details)
- Give details of telephone support lines which can provide on going support and encouragement (see the box on the adjacent page for a list of useful phone numbers)

Arrange

Monitoring progress is an essential part of successful cessation. Arranging a follow up is therefore very important. Evidence indicates that ideally patients should be initially seen 1-2 weeks after their quit date. This may fit in with a subsequent dental appointment for on going treatment or a visit to the hygienist. At this early stage people need support and encouragement. Congratulate patients who have managed not to smoke over this period. Praise and encouragement can help motivate and maintain patients determination to succeed.

Those patients who have smoked since their

Heirarchy of evidence

Type 1
Systematic review of at least one randomised controlled trial (RCT)
Type 2
At least one RCT
Type 3
Non-randomised intervention studies
Type 4
Observational studies
Type 5
Traditional reviews, expert opinion

Table 2 Potential reasons for quitting smoking

- Reduce risk of halitosis
- Improve appearance – less staining on teeth, better skin texture
- Save money
- Feel better and more energetic
- Break dependence on tobacco
- Reduced risk of cancers and heart disease
- Better periodontal health – greater chance of retaining teeth for life
- Reduced risk of oral cancers
- Improved success with surgical treatments

quit date need your support and encouragement too. Most smokers make several attempts to stop before finally succeeding. Through sensitive questioning it is important to find out what happened and any lessons that can be drawn from the experience. This will help them in future attempts to predict possible problems and increase their confidence to succeed.

Some smokers who are heavily dependent on nicotine may require more specialist and intensive support to quit. Across the country specialist smoking cessation services have been established to provide assistance to these individuals. Dentists can refer patients to these services, details of which should be available with the local Primary Care Trust or Health Promotion Service.

IMPORTANT AIDS TO SUCCESS
A range of factors make quitting smoking a difficult task for many people. One of the most important problems is the powerfully addictive nature of nicotine. Nicotine replacement therapy (NRT) can help people cope better with their cravings for nicotine, particularly moderate smokers. The use of NRT doubles a persons cessation success rate. A range of NRT products are available including patches, gums, nasal sprays, inhalators and microtabs. Recently a NRT lozenge product has also been launched. The choice of product largely depends on personal preference. NRT products have recently been made available on prescription which has helped improve access by reducing their cost, which was previously a significant barrier to their use especially amongst low income smokers.

Bupropion (Zyban), although originally developed as an anti-depressant in the US has now been licensed as a pharmaceutical treatment for tobacco dependence. A meta analysis of published trials demonstrate that the drug improves 12 month abstinence rates and reduces the severity of withdrawal symptoms.[13] The drug is available on prescription through GPs and specialist smoking clinics.

SMOKING CESSATION WORKS
The evidence base demonstrating the value of smoking cessation in primary care settings is very strong, based upon the findings of a number of randomised clinical trials.[4] Very brief advice lasting less than 3 minutes given by a health professional will help an additional 2% of smokers to successfully stop smoking each year. With more intensive support lasting up to 10 minutes, plus NRT, an additional 6% of smokers will quit.

A quit rate of 2% or even 6% may seem rather insignificant. However when translated into a population estimate, between 63,000 and 190,000 people may quit smoking each year in the UK if all general dental practitioners routinely offered smoking cessation advice based on the 4 A's model to those seeking dental care.[11] Such an impressive achievement for the dental profession can be achieved through the routine adoption of a straightforward and relatively quick protocol.

MOVING THE AGENDA FORWARDS
A range of barriers have been reported by dentists to explain the low level of routine involvement in smoking cessation activities within dental practices despite positive attitudes.[6,9,14-16] The main barriers include time and cost pressures, lack of knowledge and confidence, concerns over impact on dentist-patient relationship, doubts of the effectiveness of interventions and lack of resources for use in dental settings. How can these barriers be overcome? Table 3 outlines a variety of factors to facilitate future action.

Table 3 Facilitators for action with smoking cessation

- Reimbursement – introduction of smoking cessation fee item into GDS payment schedule
- Professional development – expansion of training opportunities in a range of topics from communication skills to knowledge of smoking treatments
- Team working – delegation of roles and responsibilities and development of team approach
- Improved communication – between staff on roles and responsibilities, with patients on relevance of oral health and smoking, and with history taking and clinical note keeping
- Multi-disciplinary working – referral of cases to specialist support when required
- Resource development – need for relevant materials for history taking and support materials for patients
- Research – need for improved evidence base on effectiveness of smoking cessation within dental settings

CONCLUSION
Smoking is the single most important public health challenge facing the NHS. The continued toll of suffering, disease and premature death resulting from tobacco use requires effective and concerted action. The government launched a national anti-smoking strategy in 1998 to co-ordinate action across the health service and beyond.[17] Dental professionals have been identified as having an important role to play in supporting smokers who desire to quit. Evidence- based guidelines provide a clear way forward for all health professionals to become engaged in this important area of prevention.[4,7] A reduction in smoking levels would improve both general and oral health,

Between 63,000 and 190,000 people may quit smoking each year in the UK if all GDPs routinely offered smoking cessation advice

Telephone support lines

Quitline
0800 00 2200
NHS Smoking Helpline
0800 169 0169
NHS Pregnancy Smoking Helpline
0800 169 9169

and would help to reduce widening inequalities across the population.

RECOMMENDATIONS ON SMOKING CESSATION WITHIN DENTAL SURGERIES

1. Tobacco use is a recognised risk factor for a host of conditions including a range of oral diseases (Type 1 Evidence).
2. Dental professionals should establish the smoking status of their patients on a regular basis (Type 3 Evidence).
3. Dental professionals should advise all smokers to stop and emphasise the oral health benefits of quitting (Type 3 Evidence).
4. Smokers who are interested and motivated to quit should be given appropriate assistance by dental professionals (Type 3 Evidence).
5. Smokers attempting to quit should be monitored and supported. Dental professionals should refer heavy smokers or those with complex needs to specialist smoking cessation services (Type 3 Evidence).

1. Callum C. *The UK smoking epidemic: Deaths in 1995.* London: Health Education Authority, 1998.
2. Legarth J, Reibel J. EU Working Group on Tobacco and Oral Health. *Oral Dis* 1998; **4:** 48-67.
3. Johnson N W, Bain C. Tobacco and oral disease. *Br Dent J* 2000; **4:** 200-206.
4. Raw M, McNeill A, West R. Smoking cessation guidelines for health professionals. A guide to effective smoking cessation interventions for the health care system. *Thorax* 1998; Suppl. **5:** 1-38.
5. Cohen S J, Stookey G K, Katz B P, Drook C A, Christen A G. Helping smokers quit: a randomised controlled trial with private practice dentists. *JADA* 1989; **118:** 41-45.
6. Smith S E, Warnakulasuriya K A A S, Feyerabend C, Belcher M, Cooper D J, Johnson N W. A smoking cessation programme conducted through dental practices in the UK. *Br Dent J* 1998; **185:** 299-303.
7. West R, McNeil A, Raw M. Smoking cessation guidelines for health professionals: an update. *Thorax* 2000; **55:** 987-999.
8. John J H, Yudkin P, Murphy M, Ziebland S, Fowler G H. Smoking cessation interventions for dental patients- attitudes and practices of dentists in the Oxford region. *Br Dent J* 1997; **183:** 359-364.
9. McCann M, Macpherson L M D, Binnie V *et al.* A survey of Scottish primary care dental practitioners' oral cancer-related practices and training requirements. *Community Dent Health* 2000; **17:** 24-30.
10. Thomas M, Walker A, Wilmot A, Bennet N. *Office for National Statistics. Living in Britain: results from the 1996 General Household Survey.* London: The Stationery Office, 1998.
11. Watt R, Robinson M. *Helping smokers to stop – a guide for the dental team.* London: Health Education Authority, 1999.
12. Warnakulasuriya K, Harris C, Scarrott D *et al.* An alarming lack of public awareness towards oral cancer. *Br Dent J* 1999; **187:** 319-322.
13. Jorenby D, Leischow S, Nides M *et al.* A controlled trial of sustained release bupropion, a nicotine patch, or both for smoking cessation. *N Eng J Med* 1999; **340:** 685-691.
14. Chestnutt I G, Binnie V I. Smoking cessation counselling-a role for the dental profession? *Br Dent J* 1995; **179:** 411-415.
15. Warnakulasuriya K A A S, Johnson N W. Dentists and oral cancer prevention in the UK: opinions, attitudes and practices of screening for mucosal lesions and to counselling patients on tobacco and alcohol use: baseline data from 1991. *Oral Dis* 1999; **5:** 10-14.
16. Allard R H B. Tobacco and oral health: attitudes and opinions of EU dentists; a report of the EU working group on tobacco and oral health. *Int Dent J* 2000; **50:** 99-102.
17. Smoking Kills: *A White Paper on Tobacco.* London: The Stationery Office, 1998.

IN BRIEF

- Nutrition plays a central role in the aetiology of a range of chronic conditions. It is essential that any dietary advice given to promote oral health is in accordance with general nutritional messages.
- Although few high quality studies have successfully altered the diet to promote oral health, evidence-based guidelines in other areas of nutrition provide a useful guide to providing dietary support in a clinical dental setting.
- The aim of this paper is to review the evidence linking diet to oral health and to outline the steps involved in providing dietary advice and support to dental patients.

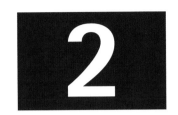

Prevention. Part 2: Dietary advice in the dental surgery

R. G. Watt[1] and P. McGlone[2]; Series Editor E. J. Kay[3]

Oral health is directly related to diet and nutrition. Dental caries remains the most significant dental public health problem in the UK and concerns have been expressed over the potentially rising prevalence of erosion. Both these conditions are linked to dietary factors. The dental professional and their teams therefore have a role to play in supporting their patients in adopting appropriate dietary habits.

PREVENTION

1. Smoking cessation advice
2. **Dietary advice**
3. **Prevention of tooth wear**
4. **Toothbrushing advice**
5. Patients requiring osseointegrated oral implant treatment
6. Older dentate patient
7. Professionally applied topical fluorides for caries prevention
8. Pit and fissure sealants in preventing caries in the permanent dentition of children

[1]*Reader, [2]Research Fellow, Department of Epidemiology and Public Health, Royal Free and University College London Medical School, University College London, 1-19 Torrington Place, London WC1E 6BT
[3]Professor of Dental Health Services Research, University of Manchester Dental Hospital and School, Higher Cambridge Street, Manchester M15 6FH
*Correspondence to: R G Watt
E-mail: r.watt@ucl.ac.uk

Reviews of oral health education and promotion interventions have highlighted the limited number of high quality studies aimed at altering diet to promote oral health.[1-5] However better quality evidence from randomised controlled trials with other primary health care professionals have highlighted the impact of dietary advice on changing dietary patterns.[6] Evidence-based guidelines now outline ways of helping patients improve their diets. This paper will provide an overview of the importance of diet on oral health and outline practical steps that can be taken within primary dental care settings to promote healthier eating patterns. The provision of dietary advice in dental practices also provides an ideal opportunity to involve and develop a team approach to patient care.

EVIDENCE ON DIET AND ORAL HEALTH

A great deal of research has been undertaken over many years into the relationship between diet and oral health. Although the totality of evidence is clear with an international scientific consensus, media coverage still frequently highlights the findings of controversial and isolated studies. As health professionals, dentists should base any advice they provide to their patients on the scientific consensus view.

Many different terms have been used to name and classify sugars. This has caused a degree of confusion amongst both the general public and health professionals. In recognition of this an expert Government committee (COMA) have recommended a revised naming system which has now become the standard classification of sugars in the UK.[7] The COMA classification is based upon where the sugar molecules are located within the food or drink structure. Intrinsic sugars are found inside the cell structure of certain unprocessed food stuffs, the most important being whole fruits and vegetables (containing mainly fructose, glucose and sucrose). Extrinsic sugars, in contrast are found outside of the cells of the food and drink. There are two types of extrinsic sugars, milk extrinsic sugars and non milk extrinsic sugars (NMES). The extrinsic milk sugars include lactose found in dairy products such as milk and milk products. NMES are found in table sugar, confectionery, soft drinks, biscuits, honey and fruit juice.

Table 1 summaries the evidence on diet and oral health based upon expert scientific reviews.[7,8]

Based upon the available evidence, consensus recommendations advocate the following points:[7,8,10,11]

- The frequency and amount of NMES should be reduced. NMES consumption should be restricted to mealtimes when possible.
- Limit consumption of NMES to a maximum of four times a day
- NMES should provide no more than 10% of total energy in the diet and not exceed 60 g per day per person
- Consumption of intrinsic sugars and starchy

Table 1 Consensus view on diet and oral health

- The influence of the diet is more important after the teeth have erupted. The pre-eruptive effect of diet on oral health is minimal.
- Non milk extrinsic sugars (NMES) are highly cariogenic.
- Frequency of eating/drinking NMES is important in caries development. However, frequency of intake and amount consumed are closely correlated.
- Intrinsic sugars eg fresh fruits and vegetables and cooked staple starchy foods such as rice and potatoes are of low cariogenicity. Milk extrinsic sugars eg milk are virtually non cariogenic.
- Alternative or non-sugar sweeteners (bulk and intense) are non-cariogenic.
- Frequent consumption of acidic drinks may be linked to the development of dental erosion

Modified from Rugg-Gunn[9]

Table 2 Eight guidelines for a healthy diet

1. Enjoy your food
2. Eat a variety of different foods
3. Eat the right amount to be a healthy weight
4. Eat plenty of foods rich in starch and fibre
5. Eat plenty of fruit and vegetables
6. Don't eat too many foods that contain a lot of fat
7. Don't have sugary foods and drinks too often
8. If you drink alcohol, drink sensibly.

Health Education Authority, 1997[12]

foods should be increased to five pieces/portions of fruit/vegetable per day.

It is essential that any dietary advice provided by dental health professionals is in accordance with general nutritional recommendations for good health (Table 2).[12,13] Oral health advice on diet must therefore not result in any increases in, for example, saturated fat intakes. In the past, well meaning oral health advice on reducing sugary snacks often resulted in an increase in fatty snacks such as crisps.

OVERVIEW OF SUGARS CONSUMPTION

Sugar has played a prominent role in British economic and political history for many centuries. In recent decades the pattern of eating in the UK has changed radically in response to wider social changes across society. From a peak in consumption in the 1950s following relaxation of war-time rationing, sugar consumption has gradually reduced. However a radical change has taken place in the pattern of consumption. There has been a large reduction in consumption of visible or table sugar (added to tea/coffee, breakfast cereals etc) and instead an increase in hidden sugars consumed in processed or manufactured foods and drinks.[14] These changes have important implications for preventive actions to promote health. Table 3 lists the sugars contents of certain popular foods and drinks.[14]

The majority of the UK population consume more NMES than the recommended 60 g/day,

although many want to reduce their intakes, often to lose weight. Particular concern focuses on the high levels of consumption amongst pre-school children, adolescents and older people. A range of barriers prevent individuals from changing what they eat (Table 4). Indeed certain groups in society have limited control over what they chose to eat. It is important for health professionals to be aware of the factors influencing their patients' dietary patterns. Taking a detailed history, setting realistic goals and monitoring any change are all essential steps in supporting patients in altering their eating habits.

EVIDENCE ON DIETARY INTERVENTIONS IN PRIMARY CARE

Very few well designed dietary interventions have been undertaken within primary dental care settings to demonstrate the effectiveness of different interventions.[1-5] This does not mean that there is no point in dentists providing dietary advice. Instead it highlights the need for better quality research into this area. Population-based interventions have shown that sugar consumption can be substantially reduced through the introduction of policy guidelines.[15] This demonstrates that sugar consumption is amenable to change given appropriate support.

A larger body of research has been undertaken to change dietary risk factors for systemic conditions such as cardiovascular disease and stroke. In a meta analysis of studies aimed at reducing dietary risk factors through advice in primary care settings, modest dietary changes were achieved which were estimated would result in a 14% reduction in CHD incidence and a 9% reduction in the incidence of stroke.[6] A systematic review of dietary interventions in primary care has highlighted characteristics of effective dietary interventions (Table 5).[16]

The challenge for the dental profession is how to translate these general guidelines into action that will facilitate a reduction in NMES consumption. The following section will outline practical steps dental practitioners and their team members can adopt to support patients adopt healthier eating patterns.

STEPS IN DIETARY COUNSELLING

Based upon evidence-based guidelines,[16] a six step model can be followed to ensure that

> As health professionals, dentists should base any dietary advice they provide to their patients on the scientific consensus view

Table 3 NMES content of popular foods and drinks

Food/Drink item	Percent NMES	Grams per serving
Coca cola regular	10.5	35.0
Ribena regular	14.0	40.0
Lucozade regular	17.9	61.8
Sunny Delight	9.8	49.0
Nestle Kit Kat	60.2	29.3
Fruit Pastilles	82.9	46.1
Kellogg's Frosties	38.0	11.2
Quaker Sugar Puffs	49.0	14.7
McVitie's Jaffa Cakes	52.0	13.0

dietary counselling is provided in a systematic and comprehensive fashion for those patients who need preventive support (Fig. 1). A clear and detailed account of each step is provided by Rugg-Gunn, and Nunn.[17]

Step 1: Identify higher risk patients

All patients should routinely be given appropriate dietary advice to maintain their oral health. For most patients this will involve a brief mention of any relevant dietary information following their clinical examination. Visual information in the form of leaflets and posters may provide reinforcement and help raise awareness of the importance of maintaining a healthy diet. For example, posters highlighting the sugar contents of popular foods and drinks may stimulate interest and motivation.

Patients with a high caries experience or evidence of erosion will require a more detailed level of support. This may apply to certain groups in particular such as pre-school children, adolescents, individuals on long-term medication and dentate older people. In addition people living in poverty may be at high risk of diet related oral health problems. Any individual at high risk of developing further oral disease should have a dietary history undertaken to determine the nature of the potential dietary problem.

Step 2: Take a dietary history

A detailed assessment of nutrient intakes is a complex, time-consuming and skilful task. Within primary dental care settings the purpose of conducting a dietary assessment is not to establish precise nutrient intakes, instead it is designed for the collection of dietary information most relevant to oral health. The key information required for this purpose is the following:

- Establishing the number of intakes per day and how many of these were snacks.
- Identifying the number of intakes that contained NMES
- Assessing whether any intakes containing NMES were taken within 1 hour of bedtime.

The most effective and feasible manner of collecting this information is through a 3-day dietary record. For three consecutive days, one of which must be on a weekend, patients are required to keep an account of all their food and drink intakes. This account should include the following information:

- Time of food or drink intake and whether eaten away from home
- Description of type of intake
- Assessment of amount of intake
- Time of going to bed

To undertake this task patients need to be very motivated and have a clear understanding of the purpose of the activity. Precise instructions on how to complete the dietary record

Table 4: Barriers to reducing NMES intakes

Individual level
- Lack of motivation to change – enjoy taste of sugary foods and drinks
- Lack of confidence to change – previous attempts have failed
- Lack of information – not clear which foods contain sugars
- Lack of skills – unable to prepare and cook healthier foods

Social level
- Peer group pressures – everyone else eats chocolate at coffee time
- Lack of time – too busy to cook
- Family pressures – husband and children will not eat vegetables
- Cultural food beliefs – sugar is needed for energy

Environmental level
- Healthier choices too costly – high costs of healthier snack foods and drinks
- Limited choices available – tuck shops only stocks soft drinks and confectionery
- Advertising pressures – children demand latest gimmick food as seen on television

Table 5 Evidence-based dietary guidelines

- Interventions should be developed from behavioural theory and should incorporate well defined goals. Information alone has only a limited impact
- Personal contact is important in motivating and monitoring change. A detailed history is required to ascertain all relevant background information
- Interventions should be tailored to individual's personal circumstances and ability to change
- Provision of feedback on dietary changes are important
- Multiple contacts over a period of time are more likely to achieve desired goals
- Encouragement and support from family and friends is essential to motivate and maintain change

Roe et al. [16]

should be given, both verbally and in a written format and the patient should be given the opportunity to ask any questions. Honesty, focus and motivation are required by the patient to complete the task accurately to avoid excessive reporting bias.

Information gathered and analysed from the diet record will provide a picture of any dietary issues that may be linked to the patient's oral health problems. Appropriate goals and an action plan can then be developed.

Step 3: Set goals

A reduction in the amount and frequency of NMES consumption is the ultimate aim of dietary advice to promote good oral health. Setting goals which are realistic (can they be achieved?), appropriate (do they take into account the individual's circumstances?) and measurable (can progress be gauged over a relatively short time frame?) are important.

Soft drinks, confectionery, and biscuits and

Fig. 1 Six step dietary counselling model

Step 1: Identify higher risk patients

Step 2: Take detailed dietary history

Step 3: Set goals

Step 4: Develop action plan

Step 5: Monitor and review

Step 6: Refer if necessary

cakes are the main sources of NMES for the majority of the population. Setting goals to reduce the consumption of these items is most likely to achieve an effect on overall NMES levels. A phased programme of reduction may help patients through a gradual alteration in their taste thresholds. Any goals need to be agreed and understood by the patient. Imposing goals on someone achieves very little.

Step 4: Develop action plan
To successfully meet agreed goals requires the development and implementation of an action plan. Dietary interventions which are tailored to the circumstances and needs of the individual are more likely to achieve desired outcomes.[18] Reviewing any past experiences in changing eating patterns may reveal useful information on ways of addressing barriers to achieving sustained changes. For example, many people report the difficulties of coping with stress and excessive pressures without resorting to chocolate or sweet eating. Discussing alternatives ways of dealing with stress could be very important.

Eating is a social activity influenced by a wide range of factors. Patients therefore need to enlist the support of their family and friends. Reflecting on the information gathered in the dietary history may identify particular times of the day when NMES are more likely to be consumed, for example, coffee breaks. Suggesting ways of altering these routines may make a real difference. Providing practical advice on alternative foods and snacks which will help reduce NMES intakes are really important (Table 6).

Table 6 Suggested foods and snacks

- Fresh fruit
- Raw vegetables
- Breadsticks
- Crackers
- Rice cakes
- Crumpets
- Currant buns, scones or teabreads
- Plain popcorn
- Savoury sandwiches, crispbreads, or pitta breads
- Water
- Milk (skimmed or semi-skimmed)
- Diluted fruit juices

Step 5: Monitor and review
With any attempt at changing behaviour, monitoring and reviewing progress is fundamentally important. There is no point spending time with a patient assessing their diet, agreeing goals and an action plan and then not seeing them again for year or so. Patients need on-going support and feedback to achieve sustained changes in their eating habits. Once an action plan has been agreed, reviewing progress within a few weeks would be ideal. Patients undergoing a course of dental treatment can have their progress assessed briefly at the end of a clinical appointment.

Step 6: Refer
In certain circumstances dietary problems may be identified which require expert guidance and support. For example, individuals who are on special diets, have a particular medical condition or have extreme dietary patterns are all beyond the expertise of dental professionals. In these cases it is best to refer the patient either to their general practitioner or a state registered dietitian for more detailed assistance. Conditions such as anorexia nervosa and bulimia may initially present with oral signs but require expert treatment and management.

TEAM APPROACH
As in any other area of clinical practice, providing dietary advice to patients is likely to be more effective when the whole dental team is actively involved.[4] Designating the appropriate roles and responsibilities of individual team members is a critical first step. Frequently due to pressures of time and in recognition of their clinical expertise, the primary role for dentists may be in the identification of patients who need dietary support and the overall co-ordination of future action. Through a detailed clinical history, dentists should be able to identify individuals who are at greatest risk from caries and erosion due to their dietary behaviour. Dentists have a professional responsibility to highlight the nature of the problem with the patient and the need for action. Delegation to appropriately trained dental nurses or hygienists for a more detailed dietary assessment and action planning may then be undertaken. Dentists however need to ensure that progress is fully monitored and reviewed at regular intervals.

CONCLUSION
Changing what people eat is not an easy task. Dentists and their team members have a responsibility however to promote and maintain the oral health of their patients. Taking a dietary history, setting appropriate and achievable goals, and developing an action plan will help patients in their attempts at controlling their sugars consumption. In addition to tailored dietary advice in the dental surgery, other public health measures aimed at the wider influences on dietary patterns are also needed to promote health and reduce inequalities across the population.

RECOMMENDATIONS: DIETARY ADVICE IN DENTAL SURGERY
1. Dietary advice should primarily aim to reduce the frequency and amount of sugary foods and drinks consumed and should be in accordance with general diet guidelines (Type 3 Evidence).
2. A dietary history should be taken to identify the pattern of sugars consumption in patients at risk of developing future caries (Type 3 Evidence).
3. Appropriate goals and an action plan should

> As in any other area of clinical practice, providing dietary advice to patients is likely to be more effective when the whole dental team is actively involved

be agreed with patients on the best means of reducing sugars consumption (Type 3 Evidence).

4. Progress with dietary changes should be monitored and reviewed. Any patients with special or complex dietary problems should be referred to their general practitioner or a state registered dietitian for detailed support (Type 3 Evidence).

1. Brown L. Research in dental health education and health promotion: a review of the literature. *Health Educ Q* 1994; **21:** 83-102.

2. Schou L, Locker D. *Oral health: A review of the effectiveness of health education and health promotion.* Amsterdam: Dutch Centre for Health promotion and Health Education, 1994.

3. Kay E J, Locker D. Is dental health education effective? A systematic review of current evidence. *Community Dent Oral Epidemiol* 1996; **24:** 231-235.

4. Sprod A, Anderson R, Treasure, E. *Effective oral health promotion. Literature Review.* Cardiff: Health Promotion Wales; 1996.

5. Kay E J, Locker D. *A systematic review of the effectiveness of health promotion aimed at promoting oral health.* London: Health Education: 1997.

6. Brunner E, White I, Thorogood M *et al.* Can dietary interventions change diet and cardiovascualr risk factors? A meta-analysis of randomised controlled trials. *Am J Public Health* 1997; **87:** 1415-1422.

7. Department of Health. *Dietary sugars and human disease.* Committee on Medical Aspects of Food Policy. London; HMSO: 1989.

8. World Health Organisation. *Diet, Nutrition and Prevention of Chronic Diseases.* Geneva: World Health Organization: 1990.

9. Rugg-Gunn A. *Nutrition and dental health.* Oxford: Oxford University Press, 1993.

10. Health Education Authority. *The scientific basis of dental health education.* A policy docment (4th Edn). London, Health Education Authority: 1996.

11. Sheiham, A. Dietary effects on dental diseases. *Public Health Nutrition* 2001; **4:** 569-591.

12. Health Education Authority. *Eight guidelines for a healthy diet. A guide for nutrition educators.* London: Health Education Authority, 1997.

13. Moynihan P J. Dietary advice in dental practice. *Br Dent J* **193:** 563-568.

14. Sustain. Sweet and sour. *The impact of sugar production and consumption on people and the environment.* London: Sustain, 2000.

15. Rodrigues C, Watt R G, Sheiham, A. The effects of dietary guidelines on sugar intake and dental caries in 3 year olds attending nurseries. *Hlth Prom Int* 1999; **14:** 329-335.

16. Roe L, Hunt P, Bradshaw H, Rayner M. H*ealth promotion interventions to promote healthy eating in the general population.* London: Health Education Authority, 1997.

17. Rugg-Gunn, A. and Nunn, J. *Nutrition, diet and oral health.* Oxford; Oxford University Press: 1999.

18. Campbell M, DeVellis B, Strecher V *et al.* Improving dietary behaviour: The effectiveness of tailored messages in primary care settings. *Am J Public Health* 1994; **84:** 783-787.

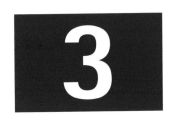

IN BRIEF

- The causes of tooth wear may be intrinsic or extrinsic and are usually chemical (acidic) or mechanical (frictional) in nature.
- Several factors may combine to cause tooth wear in any individual patient.
- Tooth wear, especially tooth erosion is an increasingly recognised clinical problem.
- Modifying the composition of soft drinks is an important concept in prevention that should be further developed.
- Although a conservative approach to restorative treatment seems justified, longitudinal clinical evaluations are needed.

Prevention. Part 3: Prevention of tooth wear

W. Peter Holbrook[1] and I. B. Árnadóttir[2]; Series Editor E. J. Kay[3]

Non-carious destruction of teeth has been observed in archaeological material from various parts of the world and clearly pre-dates the first appearance of dental caries. Attrition, abrasion and erosion are also described in the classic text of Pindborg[1] on the pathology of the dental hard tissues. Whilst the dental profession, at least in affluent parts of the world, was engaged in diagnosing, treating and later preventing dental caries these other causes of tooth destruction were largely ignored.

PREVENTION

[1]Professor, [2]Senior Lecturer, Faculty of Odontology, University of Iceland, Vatnsmýrarvegi 16, IS 101 Reykjavík, Iceland
[3]Professor of Dental Health Services Research, University of Manchester Dental Hospital and School, Higher Cambridge Street, Manchester M15 6FH
*Correspondence to: Professor W Peter Holbrook, Faculty of Odontology, University of Iceland, Vatnsmýrarvegi 16, IS 101 Reykjavik, Iceland
E-mail: phol@hi.is

Striking clinical examples of attrition were seen in patients with bruxism. Abrasion was attributed to tooth brushing or occasionally to habits such as chewing on a pipe stem. Erosion was seen in patients with symptoms of gastric reflux[2,3] and later was recognised in patients with anorexia[4] or bulimia[5] or in patients with unusual dietary habits.[6] In some cases erosion has been recognised as an occupational disease where workers have been exposed to acidic fumes, for example in factories making batteries.[7,8] It is also recognised among wine-tasters[9] (Type 4,5).

Over the past 10–15 years, however, there has been a steady increase in reports of erosion seen especially in young adults, adolescents[10] (Fig. 1) and young children as noted particularly in the UK National survey.[11] The cause of this erosion has been largely linked to the high consumption of soft drinks, both fruit juice and carbonated drinks, by these age groups. This link has been made largely in Europe and the problem has received little attention in the literature coming from the USA[12,13] (Type 4).

DIAGNOSIS AND SEVERITY

In order to prevent or reduce the non-carious destruction of tooth substance it is important first of all to:

1. Recognise that the problem is present
2. Grade its severity
3. Diagnose the likely cause or causes and,

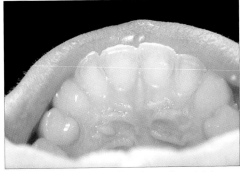

Fig. 1 Clinical appearance of erosion on the palatal surface of upper incisor teeth in a patient who consumed daily large quantities of carbonated drinks

4. Monitor progress of the disease in order to assess the success, if any, of preventive measures.

Collectively the various manifestations of non-carious tooth destruction have been termed tooth wear which conveniently allows for discussion of the problem without the obligation to meet all the precise definitions of each manifestation of the condition. Indeed many patients present with tooth wear that is the result of several aetiological factors that do not fall conveniently into one or other of the categories, attrition, abrasion or erosion (Figs 2,3). Careful observation by the dentist or hygienist at a routine visit is still probably the most usual way for tooth wear to be seen. Tooth

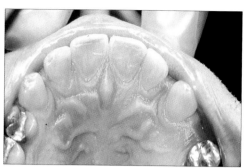

Fig. 2 Erosion on the palatal surface of maxillary incisor teeth, note the 'step' in the dentine caused by abrasion in the dentine by the lower incisors

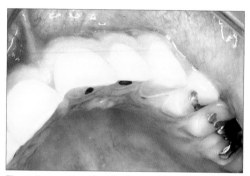

Fig. 3 Appearance of erosion in maxillary teeth of a teenage patient who consumed large quantities of carbonated drinks and also had a history of gastric reflux. Note the remains of incisal enamel at the gingival margin and erosion of the palatal cusps of the premolar and molar teeth

Frictional forces and acids cause tooth wear, singly or in combination. Although the presence of tooth wear may be obvious to the clinician, determining its cause can be difficult

wear may be present in patients with gastro-oesophageal reflux disease (Figs 4-6), bulimia and anorexia. It is clearly important for doctors and nurses treating patients with these conditions to be aware of the possibility that the patient also has severe tooth wear.

Once diagnosed, it is important that the location of the tooth wear and its severity be recorded. Several indices are available for this, ranging from the relatively simple index of Eccles and Jenkins[14] (Type 4), that was designed for recording the severity of erosion, through the more detailed modification of the same index proposed by Lussi[15] and the detailed Tooth Wear Index of Smith and Knight[16] (Type 4) that is somewhat cumbersome to use at first but gives a good record of wear on each tooth surface enabling monitoring of the progression of tooth wear. It is also not limited to tooth erosion as are most of the other indices. In epidemiological studies the degree of inter- and intra- examiner variability in detecting and scoring tooth wear may be as great a problem as determining the aetiology. Careful calibration of examiners is helpful. For an individual practitioner, clinical experience may not be sufficient for his or her purposes and even a brief examination and second opinion by a colleague may help confirm the diagnosis, its severity and possible aetiology. Study casts are clearly a useful record of the status at any particular time and can be used to monitor progression of tooth wear. Computer-aided analysis of direct imaging of the affected teeth, impressions or

study models are being developed but have not yet reached the stage of being a useful clinical tool for general practice [17,18] (Type 4). For routine clinical purposes, tooth wear should be recorded separately for the anterior and posterior teeth. The clinician should note the tooth wear as being: in enamel only; into dentine; or severely affecting the tooth or series of teeth for example as seen frequently in erosion of the palatal surfaces of four maxillary incisor teeth.

AETIOLOGY AND HISTORY TAKING

Following diagnosis of the presence of tooth wear, the clinician should attempt to determine the main aetiological factors. This will partly be based on clinical experience: examination of wear-facets; restorations that stand proud of the surrounding enamel; loss of vertical dimension; and the pattern of tooth wear. For example, a pattern of tooth wear involving the palatal surface of maxillary molar teeth, buccal surfaces of mandibular molars and palatal wear of maxillary anterior teeth is strongly suggestive of erosion caused by gastric acid. Nevertheless, other factors may play a part in the overall clinical picture. If there is a loss of occlusal enamel in the molar teeth the consequent loss of vertical dimension may produce 'step-like' wear facets palatally on the maxillary anterior teeth (Fig. 2), especially if the enamel has also been lost on these surfaces (Figs 5-6). The patient may also show other signs of more severe bruxism. A par-

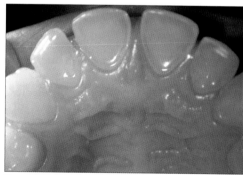

Fig. 4 Clinical appearance of maxillary anterior teeth in a patient with gastric reflux disease — note the enamel at the palatal gingival margin and the approximal surfaces

ticular diagnostic problem is the condition sometimes termed abfraction where cervical erosions occur in several teeth thought by some authors[19,20] (Type 4) to be caused by lateral occlusal forces acting in an acidic environment. These conditions may be found in a patient with bruxism who also has gastric reflux or who consumes acidic foods or beverages frequently.

Good history taking is essential to determine the consumption of carbonated drinks, fruit juices and other dietary factors that may contribute to the observed tooth wear.[15] Medication, particularly frequent use of asthma inhalers containing steroid[21,22] (Type4) or effervescent medications,[23] should be checked as they may contribute to tooth erosion. Habits, including tooth brushing, that could contribute to tooth

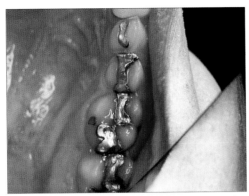

Fig. 5 Clinical appearance of maxillary posterior teeth in a patient with erosion and gastro-oesophageal reflux disease. The erosion is largely confined to the palatal aspects of these teeth

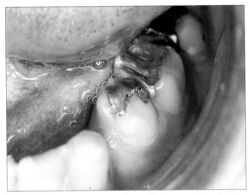

Fig. 6 Clinical appearance of mandibular posterior teeth in a patient with erosion and gastro-oesophageal reflux disease. The erosion is largely confined to the buccal aspects of these teeth

wear should be investigated with careful questions. It is important not to indicate that any blame for the clinical findings is being placed on the patient, otherwise a false history will be obtained. This is especially true when there are financial implications for the patient, for example the possibility of discretionary payments for necessary dental treatment, should the tooth wear be deemed not to be the 'fault' of the patient. The possibility of gastro-oesophageal reflux should be considered, not only bulimia and anorexia that patients are understandably reluctant to admit to, but also other possible causes of reflux including hiatus hernia.[24] It may be necessary for the dentist to refer the patient to a gastroenterologist for investigations including gastroscopy and 24-hour monitoring of oesophageal pH that is the 'gold standard' for diagnosis of gastro-oesophageal reflux disease.[25] Prompt diagnosis of reflux will in most cases lead to medication or possibly surgery to reduce reflux that will, in turn, remove the erosive challenge to the teeth (Type 4,5).

Tests of salivary function, particularly measuring salivary buffer capacity, may reveal contributing factors to tooth wear. There is no doubt that saliva plays an important role in the protection of enamel from erosion by acid, both by supplying the components of the acquired pellicle that coat the enamel surface and by promoting remineralisation of the enamel surface following acid attack. Clinical studies of the relationship between erosion and low salivary buffer capacity have, however, given conflicting results (Type 4).[25-27] Careful history taking and clinical examination bearing in mind a possible mixed aetiology of tooth wear and including questions on diet, reflux disease and functional habits should help the practitioner arrive at a correct diagnosis.

PREVENTION OF TOOTH WEAR

Preventing tooth wear is not the same as preventing caries. Dental caries is regarded as a disease that will affect most people in the world to some extent during their lifetime. This inevitability of caries developing, at least historically, was a strong stimulus to the development and promotion of preventive measures, especially those based on fluoride use and oral hygiene. Developed countries have experienced, by and large, higher prevalences of caries than less developed countries and their need for preventive measures has, therefore, been greater. Well-structured prevention programmes based on fluoride, organised dental examinations and regular recall and even financially subsidised treatments have become available that not only protect non-diseased teeth but also reduce the cariogenic challenge by removing the diseased tissue.

Tooth wear is a different and, in many ways, more difficult preventive problem. It has been regarded, until recently, as a problem for individual patients rather than being community based. With the high prevalences particularly of tooth erosion recorded in some surveys[11,28] (Type 4), it is arguable that this type of tooth wear at least has now achieved the status of a community-wide dental problem in several countries. Undoubtedly tooth wear that can be attributed to a coarse diet, to rituals such as filing down teeth and also to environmental factors can all be found in developing countries. Prevention of tooth wear in these circumstances calls for cultural and economic changes that lie outside the scope of this review.

Although tooth wear is increasingly recognised to be a problem, it is difficult to predict which individuals will be affected and true prevention is therefore difficult to achieve. Much that can now be done is aimed at limiting further tooth wear in individuals already found to be affected by this condition. Population-based strategies of prevention, such as by widespread modification of the composition of soft drinks and educational campaigns to increase awareness of the causes of tooth wear may be possible but it is not likely that they will meet with the widespread acceptance that preventive strategies for caries have achieved. This is in part due to the age group perceived to be most at risk of developing erosion, teenagers and young adults, being rather resistant to the messages of health educators, at least when the message relates to reducing the consumption of erosive drinks that

Although tooth wear is now a community-wide problem, population-based preventive strategies will probably be less effective than for dental caries

are so much a part of the lifestyle of this age group. More can possibly be done with an at-risk strategy aimed at specific individuals with early signs of tooth wear or with known risk factors for tooth wear present, such as those taking medicines known to be erosive and patients with bulimia. For such a strategy to work collaboration between the dentist and other healthcare professionals is important.

PREVENTIVE STRATEGIES

Strategies for preventing tooth wear are largely based on the individual. Abrasion and attrition are disorders that are individual-based. Erosion has certain features, including its prevalence and relationship to diet, that make the disease problem somewhat similar to that of caries. Few, if any, population-based strategies that have been so successful in caries prevention have, however, been shown to have an effect on erosion. The perceived increase in the prevalence of tooth erosion has produced an upsurge of research into possible ways of preventing erosion whereas other forms of tooth wear have received less attention.

Fluoride

Fluoride is the mainstay of caries prevention and it was, therefore, natural for fluoride to be considered as a possible vehicle for preventing tooth erosion. In fact the literature contains conflicting reports about the benefits of fluoride in this respect. A number of animal and in vitro studies suggest that adding fluoride to potentially erosive drinks will reduce the erosive potential of these drinks.[29-31] Addition of fluoride to sports drinks has also been shown to reduce the erosive potential of these, otherwise highly erosive, drinks.[32] Amaechi et al.,[33] have shown that xylitol and fluoride have an additive effect in reducing the erosive potential of orange juice in in vitro studies. Larsen,[34] however, showed that the protective effect against erosion of fluoride added to soft drinks was minimal. Clearly some more research is required in this area to resolve these differences, perhaps through the development of agreed test systems to evaluate erosive potential. It is known that tooth brushing shortly after drinking an erosive beverage causes an increase in tooth wear. Topical fluoride appears to protect against this subsequent tooth wear following acid challenge.[35-37] This is especially helpful in reducing dentine wear in previously eroded teeth.[38] Fluoride, therefore, appears to have only a limited protective effect against erosive challenge in vivo (Type 4).

Drink modification

Drink modification has been developing in recent years with varying success.[30] Addition of calcium lactate to Coca Cola® has been shown to reduce the erosive potential of this most international of erosive beverages[39] but this research does not appear to have been taken up by the manufacturer. Rather the reverse trend is seen with the marketing of drinks with added citric

acid to drinks such as Pepsi Cola® and to several diet preparations of carbonated drinks. This increases the erosive potential of these drinks, at least when measured in vitro.[40] A successful attempt to reduce the erosive potential of soft drinks by the addition of calcium citrate-malate was reviewed by Grenby[30] but a later in vivo investigation by Rugg-Gunn et al.[41] found no difference in the amount of erosion seen in enamel slabs treated with plain or modified orange drinks. One of the potentially most important steps in soft drink modification has been the development and subsequent marketing of Ribena Tooth Kind.[42-44] This low pH blackcurrant drink has been modified with the addition of calcium and has been shown in in situ and in vitro studies to be less erosive than blackcurrant drinks without added calcium and also less erosive than orange juice. Considering the increasing prevalence of tooth erosion, especially in young children and teenagers and the strong association between consumption of acidic drinks and tooth erosion, it still seems logical to continue the development of drinks with low erosive potential. Drink modification has considerable potential in combating erosion but clinical trials are needed.

Diet modification is a difficult area in which to achieve successful disease prevention as experience from dental caries has shown. Nevertheless the strong links between dietary factors and tooth wear make it sensible for the dental team to at least try to get patients with tooth wear to modify their diet. Patients with tooth wear thought to be linked to dietary acids should be closely questioned about their dietary habits and modifications, suggested including reducing the frequency of consumption of these foods limiting consumption of fruit and fruit juices to mealtimes. Consuming hard cheese or milk products after drinking an erosive beverage may promote re-hardening of the enamel[45,46] (Type 4). This is probably also a useful method of neutralising acid in the mouth after a bout of reflux or vomiting but patient compliance is perhaps questionable. Chewing-gum containing carbamide (urea) has been shown to raise salivary pH rapidly[47] (Type 4). This may, therefore, reduce the erosive effect of acid in the mouth.

The pattern of drinking erosive beverages is thought to contribute to tooth erosion[48] (Type 4) especially when cola-type drinks are swished around the mouth before swallowing. Drinking through a straw has been shown to reduce the potential for tooth erosion from acidic drinks[49] (Type 4), especially on the palatal surfaces of the maxillary incisors that are most commonly affected in patients with erosion.

Abrasion caused by diet or tothbrushing is greater if the teeth have been recently exposed to dietary or gastric acid. It has been shown by Attin et al.[50] that resistance to this abrasion develops in the mouth but that at least 60 min should elapse after an acid challenge to the teeth before brushing. This is probably of particular significance for patients who have frequent

Modifying drinks to make them less erosive is still the most promising and realistic preventive measure against tooth erosion

episodes of vomiting but it is also sensible for dentists to advise their patients not to brush shortly after consuming carbonated drinks. Similarly, mouthrinses with a low pH should not be recommended for prolonged use nor as pre-brushing rinses.[51] Remineralizing toothpaste (Enamelon™) has been shown to increase the hardness of acid-treated teeth significantly more than conventional fluoride toothpastes in *in vitro* studies.[52]

Saliva and pellicle are important factors in protection of tooth substance against acid attack. Amaechi *et al.*[33] and Johansson *et al.*[47] have shown that erosion is usually found in areas of the dental arches that are lacking in pellicle. Increasing salivary flow and hence accumulation of pellicle will, therefore, probably offer protection against erosion. Data from clinical trials are lacking, however, although Hall *et al.*[53] (Type 4) have demonstrated this protective effect of salivary pellicle in an *in-situ* model system. Increasing salivary flow and, consequently, buffer capacity should increase protection against erosion and promote remineralization. Sugar-free chewing gum and even fluoride-containing or carbamide-containing gum should be advised, particularly for adolescents who may be least willing to limit their consumption of acidic beverages. A number of preparations intended to promote salivation are available for patients including those with dry mouth symptoms who may not be willing to chew gum. Profylin™ (Prophylactor AB, Sweden) and Xerodent™ (Dumex-Alpharma, Denmark) lozenges are examples of such topical preparations and Xerodent™ has the added advantage of containing fluoride.

Gastric reflux

Reflux disease and vomiting are important causes of tooth erosion. Recognition of the erosion and presumptive diagnosis by the dentist should lead to appropriate referral for further investigation. Most often this will be to a gastroenterologist for gastroscopy and for 24-hour measurements of oesophageal pH. Medication to reduce gastric reflux and acid production includes drugs such as over-the-counter antacids or prescription drugs such as omeprazolum (Losec®) and ranitidinum (Asyran®). Should hiatus hernia be diagnosed then surgical intervention may be necessary. Diagnosis and treatment of the underlying condition is obviously a pre-requisite to stopping the progression of the tooth wear. In many cases of tooth wear associated with gastric disturbance, both attrition and erosion are seen. Because many individuals with erosion are young males, in our clinical experience at least, they are in the age group that is known to consume a lot of acidic drink but this is also the age group that is active in sport and training and may, for example experience gastric reflux as a consequence (Holbrook *et al.* unpublished findings, Type 4). Diagnosis of the tooth wear may be clear but determining the aetiological factors involved may, however, be difficult.[54] Should the dentist believe that the patient may have bulimia then referral to a psychiatrist may be indicated. This is often difficult and depends to a great extent on the rapport and trust that the dentist has built up with the patient. At the very least the dentist should convey his suspicion to the patient's general medical practitioner. Careful monitoring of the progress of the tooth wear over time, for example with study casts, is helpful both for the dentist and as an aid to increase patient cooperation. The use of fluoride and antacid medications as well as the protective effect of cheese should be emphasised and careful instruction on tooth brushing technique to minimise abrasion should be given (Type 5).[55]

Lifestyle changes

Lifestyle changes are particularly difficult to achieve, especially in the age groups that are frequently found to have tooth wear. Drinking carbonated beverages with a straw; eating a piece of cheese shortly afterwards; and taking antacids,[56] xylitol gum or xylitol-fluoride-containing lozenges[57] after exercise are not activities that fit in particularly well with the lifestyle of young people. Nevertheless the dental profession has the responsibility to inform patients of the problem and its consequences. The success of fluoride in preventing dental caries in populations that continue to consume sugar at high levels is not likely to be repeated with tooth erosion. Indeed the rise in awareness of tooth erosion, in Europe at least, has occurred as caries levels have rapidly declined. Whether or not modification of acidic drinks to make them less erosive will prove possible or even acceptable to manufacturers and public alike remains to be seen. Considerable financial sums are at stake for the industry and it seems unlikely that these will be risked without public demand or legislation.

Restorative procedures

Restorative treatment of teeth affected by tooth wear is very expensive and not always covered by health services, even in Europe. There is also still a need for long-term studies on tooth wear, particularly into how erosion and related tooth wear progresses in young people. This makes authoritative recommendations on restorative measures impossible until further research has been completed. Various non-or minimally-invasive procedures have been tried in order to prevent further tooth wear but clearly extensive crown and bridge work is sometimes required. Lambrechts *et al.*[58] have reviewed the various therapeutic approaches and point out that the durability of crown and bridgework is only 15–20 years which should be borne in mind in the light of the age group frequently presenting in the dental surgery with tooth wear. Conservative approaches that may also offer a degree of protection/prevention against further wear are therefore urgently sought as are restorative techniques that do not involve further destruction of remaining tooth substance. Dentine-

Tooth wear may be an indication of underlying reflux disease or bulimia. Collaboration between medical and dental practitioners is important in treating such cases

PREVENTION

Restorative procedures that do not involve yet more destruction of tooth substance should be attempted. More research in this area is needed

bonding agents have been shown to be effective in reducing sensitivity and offering protection against further dissolution of erosive lesions[59,60] (Type 3). These should be applied and the patient monitored before any final decision is taken on restorative measures.[55]

Prevention of attrition and abrasion is not usually considered until the patient actually has signs of the problem. Diagnosis is usually more straightforward than with erosion except in cases where attrition or abrasion are superimposed on erosion when diagnosis can become problematical. Patients with bruxism may well need occlusal splints, at least to use at night, and restorative treatment is frequently necessary. Correction of tooth brushing technique and the use of less abrasive toothpaste should help reduce abrasion and habits that may lead to abrasion should be controlled. As with tooth erosion it is helpful to make study casts and to monitor progression of the tooth wear.

CONCLUSION

A considerable increase in tooth wear has been observed in recent years. This is predominantly erosion though often complicated by other forms of tooth wear. Careful diagnosis and monitoring of progress are important and the underlying aetiological factors should be corrected wherever possible. The aetiology of tooth wear is often complex but individualised prevention can usually only be initiated once the disease has started. This is largely aimed at limiting progression of tooth wear in the affected individual. Population-based strategies are largely inappropriate in preventing tooth wear although modification of erosive drinks, medicines and foods may prove to be an acceptable future strategy for manufacturer and customer alike. Careful monitoring of patients following diagnosis of tooth wear, removal of causative factors and relatively simple dental treatments may enable the patient to avoid extensive restorative procedures.

1. Pindborg J J. *Pathology of the dental hard tissues.* Copenhagen: Munksgaard 1970.
2. Järvinen V, Meurman J H, Hyvärnen H, Rytömaa I, Murtomaa H. Dental erosion and upper gastrointestinal disorders. *Oral Surg Oral Med Oral Pathol* 1988; **65**; 298-303.
3. Meurman J, Toskala J, Nuutinen P, Klemetti E. Oral and dental manifestations in gastroesophageal reflux disease. *Oral Surg Oral Med Oral Pathol* 1994; **78**: 583-589.
4. Hellström I. Anorexia nervosa-odontologiska problem. *Swed Dent J* 1974; **67**: 253-269.
5. Trygstad O. Bulimi-et liv uten kontroll. *Nord Med* 1986; **101**: 72-77.
6. Linkosalo E, Markanen S. Dental erosions in relation to lactovegetarian diet. *Scand J Dent Res* 1989; **93**: 436-441.
7. Petersen P E, Gormsen C. Oral conditions among German battery factory workers. *Community Dent Oral Epidemiol* 1991; **19**: 104-106.
8. Tuominen M, Tuominen R. Dental erosion and associated factors among factory workers exposed to inorganic acid fumes. *Proc Finn Dent Soc* 1991; **87**: 359-364.
9. Gray A, Ferguson M M, Wall J G. Wine tasting and dental erosion. Case report. *Aust Dent J* 1998; **43**: 32-34.
10. Lussi A, Schaffner M, Hotz P, Sutter P. Dental erosion in a population of Swiss adults. *Community Dent Oral Epidemiol* 1991; **19**: 286-290.
11. Downer M C. The 1993 national survey of children's dental health. *Br Dent J* 1995; **178**: 407-412.
12. Bartlett D, Phillips K, Smith B. A difference in perspective – the North American and European interpretations of tooth wear. *Int J Prosthodont* 1999; **12**: 401-408.
13. Deery C, Wagner M L, Longbottom C, Simon R, Nugent Z J. The prevalence of dental erosion in a United States and a United Kingdom sample of adolescents. *Pediatr Dent* 2000; **22**: 505-510.
14. Eccles J D, Jenkins W G. Dental erosion and diet. *J Dent* 1974; **2**: 153-159.
15. Lussi A. Dental erosion : clinical diagnosis and history taking. *Eur J Oral Sci* 1996; **104**: 191-198.
16. Smith B G, Knight J K. An index for measuring the wear of teeth. *Br Dent J* 1984; **156**: 435-438.
17. Hall A F, Sadler J P, Strang R, de Josselin de Jong E, Foye R H, Creanor S L. Application of transverse microradiography for measurement of mineral loss by acid erosion. *Adv Dent Res* 1997; **11**: 420-425.
18. Azzopardi A, Bartlett D W, Watson T F, Smith B G. A literature review of the techniques to measure tooth wear and erosion. *Eur J Prosthodont Restor Dent* 2000; **8**: 93-97.
19. Grippo J O, Simring M. Dental 'erosion' revisited. *J Am Dent Assoc* 1995; **126**: 619-630.
20. Rees J S. A review of the biomechanics of abfraction. *Eur J Prosthodont Restor Dent* 2000; **8**: 139-144.
21. Al-Dlaigan Y H, Shaw L, Smith A J. Is there a relationship between asthma and dental erosion? A case control study. *Int J Paediatr Dent* 2002; **12**: 189-200.
22. O'Sullivan E A, Curzon M E. Drug treatments for asthma may cause erosive tooth damage. *Br Med J* 1998; **317**: 820.
23. Nunn J H, Ng S K, Sharkey I, Coulthard M. The dental implications of chronic use of acidic medicines in medically compromised children. *Pharm World Sci* 2001; **23**: 118-119.
24. Scheutzel P. Etiology of dental erosion-intrinsic factors. *Eur J Oral Sci* 1996; **104**: 178-190.
25. Gudmundsson K, Kristleifsson G, Theodors A, Holbrook P. Tooth erosion, gastroesophageal reflux and salivary buffer capacity. *Oral Surg Oral Med Oral Pathol Oral Radiol Endod* 1995; **79**: 185-189.
26. Bevenius J, L'Estrange P. Chairside evaluation of salivary parameters in patients with tooth surface loss: a pilot study. *Aust Dent J* 1990; **35**: 219-221.
27. Wöltgens J, Vingerling P, de Blieck-Hogervorst, Bervoets D. Enamel erosion and saliva. *Clin Prev Dent* 1985; **7**: 8-10.
28. Milosevic A, Young PJ, Lennon M A. The prevalence of tooth wear in 14-year-old school children in Liverpool. *Community Dent Hlth* 1993; **11**: 83-86.
29. Holloway P J, Mellanby M, Stewart R J C. Fruit drinks and tooth erosion. *Br Dent J* 1958; **104**: 305-309.
30. Grenby T H. Lessening dental erosive potential by product modification. *Eur J Oral Sci* 1996; **104**: 221-228.
31. Ganss C, Klimek J, Schaffer U, Spall T. Effectiveness of two fluoridation measures on erosion progression in human enamel and dentine *in vitro. Caries Res* 2001; **35**: 325-330.
32. Sorvari R, Kiviranta I, Luoma H. Erosive effect of a sport drink mixture with and without addition of fluoride and magnesium on the molar teeth of rats. *Scand J Dent Res* 1988; **96**: 226-231.
33. Amaechi B T, Higham S M, Edgar W M, Milosevic A. Thickness of acquired salivary pellicle as a determinant of the sites of dental erosion. *J Dent Res* 1999; **78**: 1821-1828.
34. Larsen M J. Prevention by means of fluoride of enamel erosions as caused by soft drinks and orange juice. *Caries Res* 2001; **35**: 229-234.
35. Sorvari R, Meurman J H, Alakuijala P, Frank R M. Effect of fluoride varnish and solution on enamel erosion *in vitro. Caries Res* 1994; **28**: 227-232.
36. Bartlett D W, Smith B G, Wilson R F. Comparison of the effect of fluoride and non-fluoride toothpaste on tooth wear in vitro and the influence of enamel fluoride concentration and hardness of enamel. *Br Dent J* 1994; **176**: 346-348.
37. Attin T, Deifuss H, Hellwig E. Influence of acidified fluoride gel on abrasion resistance of eroded enamel. *Caries Res* 1999; **33**: 135-139.
38. Attin T, Zirkel C, Hellwig E. Brushing abrasion of eroded dentin after application of sodium fluoride solutions. *Caries Res* 1998; **32**: 344-350.
39. Beiraghi S, Atkins S, Rosen S, Wilson S, Odom J, Beck M. Effect of calcium lactate in erosion and *S.mutans* in rats when added to Coca-Cola. *Pediatr Dent* 1989; **11**: 312-315.
40. Jensdottir T. *Dental erosion and beverages-clinical and laboratory investigation.* Thesis. Reykjavik: University of Iceland 2002;pp33-44 (ISBN 9979-9525-0-4)
41. Rugg-Gunn A J, Maguire A, Gordon P H, McCabe J F, Stephenson G. Comparison of erosion of dental enamel by

four drinks using an intra-oral appliance. *Caries Res* 1998; **32:** 337-343.

42. Hughes J A, West N X, Parker D M, Newcombe R G, Addy M. Development and evaluation of a low erosive blackcurrant juice drink *in vitro* and *in situ*. 1. Comparison with orange juice. *J Dent* 1999a; **27:** 285-289.
43. Hughes J A, West N X, Parker D M, Newcombe R G, Addy M. Development and evaluation of a low erosive blackcurrant juice drink. 3. Final drink and concentrate, formulae comparisons in situ and overview of the concept. *J Dent* 1999b; **27:** 354-350.
44. West N X, Hughes J A, Parker D M, Newcombe R G, Addy M. Development and evaluation of a low erosive blackcurrant juice drink. 2. Comparison with a conventional blackcurrant juice drink and orange juice. *J Dent* 1999; **27:** 341-344.
45. Gedalia I, Dakuar A, Shapira L, Lewinstein I, Goultschin J, Rahmim E. Enamel softening with Coca-cola and rehardening with milk or saliva. *Am J Dent* 1991; **4:** 120-122.
46. Gedalia I, Davidov I, Lewinstein I Shapira L. Effect of hard cheese exposure with and without fluoride prerinse on the rehardening of softened human enamel. *Caries Res* 1992; **26:** 290-292.
47. Imfeld T, Birkhed D, Lingström P. Effect of urea in sugar-free chewing gums on pH recovery in human dental plaque evaluated with three different methods. *Caries Res* 1995; **29:** 172-180.
48. Johansson A-K, Lingström P, Birkhed D. Comparison of factors potentially related to the occurrence of dental erosion in high- and low- erosion groups. *Eur J Oral Sci* 2002; **110:** 204-211.
49. Edwards M, Ashwood R A, Littlewood S J, Brocklebank L M, Fung D E. A videofluoroscopic comparison of straw and cup drinking: the potential influence on dental erosion. *Br Dent J* 1998; **185:** 244-249.
50. Attin T, Knofel S, Buchalla W, Tutuncu R. *In situ* evaluation of different remineralization periods to decrease brushing

abrasion of demineralised enamel. *Caries Res* 2001; **35:** 216-222.
51. Pontefract H, Hughes J, Kemp K, Yates R, Newcombe RG, Addy M The erosive effects of some mouthrinses on enamel. A study *in situ*. *J Clin Periodontol* 2001; **28:** 319-324.
52. Munoz C A, Feller R, Haglund A, Triol C W, Winston A E. Strengthening of tooth enamel by a remineralizing toothpaste after exposure to an acidic soft drink. *J Clin Dent* 1999; **10** (1 Spec no):17-21.
53. Hall A F, Buchanan C A, Millett D T, Creanor S L, Strang R, Foye RH. The effect of saliva on enamel and dentine erosion. *J Dent* 1999; **27:** 333-339.
54. Bartlett D W, Coward P Y, Nikkah C, Wilson R F. The prevalence of tooth wear in a cluster sample of adolescent schoolchildren and its relationship with potential explanatory factors. *Br Dent J* 1998; **184:** 125-129.
55. Sundram G, Bartlett D. Preventive measures for bulimic patients with dental erosion. *Eur J Prosthodont Restor Dent* 2001; **9:** 25-29.
56. Meurman J H, Kuittinen T, Kanga M, Tuisku T. Buffering effect of antacids in the mouth- a new treatment of dental erosion? *Scand J Dent Res* 1988; **96:** 412-417.
57. Tenovuo J, Hurme T, Ahola A, Svedberg C, Ostela I, Lenander-Lumikari M, Neva M. Release of cariostatic agents from a new buffering fluoride- and xylitol-containing lozenge to human whole saliva *in vivo*. *J Oral Rehabil* 1997; **24:** 325-331.
58. Lambrechts P, Van Meerbeek B, Perdigao J, Gladys S, Braem M, Vanherle G. Restorative therapy for erosive lesions. *Eur J Oral Sci* 1996; **104:** 229-240.
59. Brunton P A, Kalsi K S, Watts D C, Wilson N H. Resistance of two dentin-bonding agents and a dentin desensitizer to acid erosion *in vitro*. *Dent Mater* 2000; **16:** 351-355.
60. Azzopardi A, Bartlett D W, Watson T F, Sheriff M. The measurement and prevention of erosion and abrasion. *J Dent* 2001; **29:** 395-400.

IN BRIEF

- Clinicians have an important role in advising patients about toothbrushing. By modifying this well accepted habit significant increases in health benefit can be gained.
- Caries reductions can be increased by increasing brushing frequency, using higher concentration fluoride formulations and limiting rinsing
- Periodontal disease can be controlled by teaching effective twice daily brushing, advising the correct design brush and toothpaste.

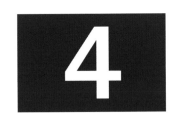

Prevention. Part 4: Toothbrushing : What advice should be given to patients?

R. M. Davies[1], G. M. Davies[2] and R. P. Ellwood[3]; Series Editor E. J. Kay[4]

This paper examines and summarises the evidence to support the advice that GDPs should give their patients on toothbrushing. The strength of evidence is graded using a five-point hierarchical scale. Much of the evidence to support toothbrushing advice is relatively weak but the increasing number of high quality systematic reviews will gradually improve the strength of evidence to support effective programmes of preventive care. Clinicians can play an important role in maximising the benefits of toothbrushing with fluoride toothpaste for patients of all ages. This well-accepted health behaviour can, if implemented correctly, reduce the establishment and advance of the two major dental diseases.

[1]Director, [3]Technology Manager, Dental Health Unit, Manchester, UK; [2]Senior Dental Officer (Epidemiology), Central Manchester Primary Care Trust, Manchester [4]Professor of Dental Health Services Research, University of Manchester Dental Hospital and School, Higher Cambridge Street, Manchester M15 6FH
Correspondence to: R. M. Davies, Dental Health Unit, Manchester Science Park, Lloyd Street North, Manchester M15 6SH
E-mail: robin.davies@man.ac.uk

Twice daily brushing with a fluoride toothpaste has been widely promoted by the profession for many years since it plays a pivotal role in the prevention and control of dental caries and periodontal diseases. Such behaviour, although self-reported, appears to be an integral part of many people's daily hygiene routine. In Great Britain 55% of children aged 1.5 to 4.5 years were reported to have their teeth brushed more than once a day[1] and in the UK 64% of 4 to18 year olds[2] and 74% of dentate adults claimed to brush their teeth twice a day.[3] Whilst it is generally accepted that such behaviour has been the most important contributor to the improvement in the dental health of the nation a sizeable proportion of the population still do not even claim to brush twice daily.

Contrary to the prevailing view that caries is under control the disease poses a potential threat throughout the lifetime of the individual. In a recent longitudinal study of 2,293 regularly attending adults, a total of 3,030 teeth (37% of those that received treatment during the 5 years) were treated for caries.[4] The increasing dentate elderly population are particularly vulnerable; 29% of dentate adults, aged 65+, had root caries with an average of 2.3 teeth affected.[5]

In the UK, the prevalence of plaque and periodontal disease also remains high;[3] 72 % of dentate adults and 33% of teeth had visible plaque and 54% of adults had pocketing greater than 3.5 mm. Although severe periodontal disease is relatively uncommon, with only 8% of dentate

adults having loss of attachment of 6 mm or more, this increased to 31% in those aged 65 and over. It was concluded that if large numbers of teeth are to be retained into old age there is a need to improve the oral cleanliness of the majority of the UK population.[6]

A search was made to identify systematic reviews on the Cochrane Library, DARE and Medline. A further search of Medline using 'toothbrush*' as a free text term produced a vast list of publications too numerous to assess. A number of symposia which had reviewed relevant topics and provided consensus statements were sourced. The last search was conducted in June 2002. Using the data from these different sources we have made recommendations as to the advice dental professionals should give their patients about toothbrushing. The strength of evidence to support each recommendation will be indicated using the following hierarchy of evidence:

Type 1 Systematic review of at least one randomised controlled trial (RCT)
Type 2 At least one RCT
Type 3 Non-randomised intervention studies
Type 4 Observational studies
Type 5 Traditional reviews, expert opinion

Randomised controlled trials are accepted as the most robust study design but they may not be ethical or practical to undertake in certain areas. For example, observational studies have provided data on the reported frequency of toothbrushing and rinsing behaviour and should not be undervalued.

CARIES

The role of oral hygiene
The ubiquitous use of fluoride toothpaste makes it difficult to distinguish whether the effect of toothbrushing on caries is the result of the mechanical removal of plaque or a measure of fluoride application.[7] Clearly the caries predilection sites, ie. occlusal pits and fissures and approximal surfaces are the most difficult to clean with toothbrush and toothpaste and traditional reviews (Type 5) of the literature have generally concluded that the effect of oral cleanliness *per se* on caries is equivocal.[8,9] Prior to the widespread availability of fluoride toothpastes, evidence of the relative importance of oral hygiene and fluoride was provided by a 3-year study (Type 2) in which two groups of children, aged 9–11 years, had supervised brushing with or without a fluoride toothpaste whilst a control group received no supervision.[10] Both the supervised brushing groups had significantly reduced plaque and gingivitis scores when compared with the control group but a significant reduction in dental caries was only observed in the fluoride toothpaste group. It is generally accepted that the decline in dental caries can be attributed, primarily, to fluoride toothpaste[11] and it would now be considered unethical to withhold the benefits of this from any group in a clinical trial.

Conclusion: The evidence that brushing *per se* is important in the prevention and control of caries is equivocal.

Evidence: Type 5

FLUORIDE TOOTHPASTE
It is generally accepted that the beneficial effects of fluoride toothpaste on dental caries are due to the topical effect of fluoride once the teeth have erupted. In contrast, the risk of fluorosis is due to the unintentional swallowing of toothpaste during tooth development. The parents of children less than 7 years should be strongly advised to apply only a small amount of toothpaste (pea or smear) and encourage the child to spit out.

A recent Cochrane Review (Type 1) concluded that the use of fluoride toothpaste is associated, on average, with a 24% reduction of dental caries in the permanent dentition of children and adolescents when compared with a non-fluoride toothpaste.[12] The effect of fluoride toothpaste on the deciduous dentition was limited to one study, which reported a reduction of 37% when compared with a non-fluoride toothpaste.

Frequency of brushing
The effectiveness of brushing twice daily with a fluoride toothpaste on caries is supported by data on reported behaviour (Type 4) obtained from surveys[1,3] and clinical trials.[13,14] For example, among children aged 3.5–4.5 years, 24% of those whose teeth were brushed more than once a day had caries experience compared

with 38% of those whose teeth were brushed once a day and almost half (48%) of those whose teeth were brushed less often.[1] In clinical trials the 3-year caries increments in participants who reported brushing only once a day were 20–30% more than those who brushed twice a day.[13,14] Whilst these data need to be interpreted with some caution because of associations with other confounding factors, such as social class and sugar consumption, the weight and consistency of available evidence supports the recommendation that toothbrushing, with a fluoride toothpaste, should be performed twice daily.[15]

Recommendation: Brush twice daily with a fluoride toothpaste.
Evidence: (Type 4,5)

Fluoride concentration
In Europe, toothpastes containing a maximum fluoride concentration of 1500 ppm are on general sale as cosmetic products. Formulations with higher concentrations are available as prescription only medicines.

An extensive review (Type 5) of clinical trials of fluoride toothpastes indicated that fluoride concentration is an important determinant of anticaries efficacy.[16] Overall, the results suggest that within the range 1000 to 2500 ppm F each increase of 500 ppm F provides an additional 6% reduction in caries.[17]

Low fluoride toothpastes, containing less than 600 ppm F, are available for young children in the UK. A recent systematic review[18] concluded that toothpastes containing 250 ppm F were not as effective at preventing caries in the permanent dentition as toothpastes containing 1000 ppm F or more (Type 1). Clinical trials in pre-school children (Type 2) comparing 550 ppm F with 1055 ppm F[19]and 440 ppm F with 1450 ppm F[20] have demonstrated that toothpastes containing the lower concentrations of fluoride provide less protection than those containing higher concentrations.

A number of randomised clinical trials[21,22] have reported that toothpastes containing fluoride concentrations higher than 1500 ppm F provide greater protection than toothpastes containing conventional levels of fluoride. Such a high fluoride toothpaste, containing 2800 ppm F, has been launched recently as a prescription only toothpaste for high caries risk individuals over 16 years of age and particularly the elderly.

Recommendation: The appropriate fluoride concentration to recommend for an individual should be made after assessing their caries risk. This should involve an assessment of previous caries experience, the most powerful predictor of future caries[23,24] together with a consideration of family history and socio-economic status.

A low fluoride concentration toothpaste (< 600 ppm F) is appropriate for low caries risk children, less than 7 years of age, particularly if living in a fluoridated area.

A toothpaste containing a higher concentration of fluoride (1000-1450 ppm F) is appropriate for high caries risk children less than 7 years

There is strong evidence that twice daily brushing with fluoride toothpaste is effective in reducing oral caries

of age with the proviso that the parent applies only a pea-sized amount or smear to the toothbrush.

A high fluoride toothpaste (1450 ppm F) can be recommended for all individuals 7 years of age or older.

A toothpaste containing 2800 ppm F is appropriate for high caries risk adults and the elderly.

Evidence: (Type 1, 2)

Rinsing behaviour

An important determinant of anticaries efficacy of a fluoride toothpaste is the rinsing behaviour after brushing. The volume of water used and the vigour of rinsing after toothbrushing affect the fluoride concentration in the mouth and caries experience.[25-27] Individuals should be advised not to rinse or to do so briefly with a small amount of water. Young children should be encouraged simply to spit out any excess toothpaste.

Recommendation: Discourage rinsing with large volumes of water. Encourage young children to spit out excess toothpaste.

Evidence: (Type 4,5)

Amount of toothpaste

Data concerning the effect that the amount of toothpaste has on efficacy is sparse. One clinical trial (Type 2) of dentifrices containing 1000, 1500 and 2500 ppm F reported that the fluoride concentration was more important than the amount of toothpaste applied.[28] Since very young children may swallow a large amount of toothpaste,[29,30] thereby increasing the risk of fluorosis, parents should supervise very young children and place only a small amount of toothpaste[31]

(smear or pea size) on the brush. It is important to reinforce this advice since 31% of children aged 1.5 to 4.5 were reported to always brush their own teeth and 45% covered half the length of the brush or more.[1]

Recommendation: Toothbrushing by children should be supervised and only a smear or pea sized amount of toothpaste should be used.

Evidence: (Type 2,4,5)

When to brush

There is no evidence to indicate the relative anti-caries benefits of brushing before or after eating meals. Recent surveys have reported that 61% of 1.5–4.5 year olds brush after breakfast and 52% last thing at night[1] for adults the values were 46% and 74% respectively.[3] However, recent evidence (Type 4) supports a recommendation that brushing with a fluoride toothpaste should take place just prior to going to bed; fluoride concentrations in saliva 12 hours after brushing last thing at night were comparable with those found 1–4 hours after brushing during the day.[32]

Recommendation: Brush last thing at night and on one other occasion.

Evidence: (Type 4,5)

Type of fluoride

There is some controversy regarding the comparative efficacy of the two major types of fluoride used in toothpastes; sodium fluoride (NaF) and sodium monofluorophosphate (MFP). A systematic review (Type 1) suggested that NaF was superior to MFP[33] but this was disputed.[34] If any difference does exist between these two species it is unlikely to be of any clinical significance. Toothpastes containing either fluoride species can be recommended with confidence.

> The effectiveness of fluoride toothpaste is influenced by frequency, concentration and rinsing behaviour; frequency having the greatest impact

Table 1 The levels of evidence for recommendations for caries control

	Instructions	Evidence
Frequency of brushing	Brush twice a day with a fluoride toothpaste.	Type 4,5
Fluoride concentration	The choice of fluoride concentration should be based on the age and perceived caries risk of the individual and their exposure to other fluoride sources. A low fluoride concentration toothpaste (< 600 ppm F) is appropriate for low caries risk children, < 7 years of age, particularly if living in a fluoridated area. A high fluoride toothpaste (1450 ppm F) is appropriate for high caries risk, < 7 years of age, with the proviso that the parent applies only a pea sized amount or smear to the toothbrush. Such a concentration can be recommended to all individuals over 6 years of age. A toothpaste containing 2800 ppm F is appropriate for high caries risk adults and the elderly.	Type 1,2
Amount of toothpaste	Toothbrushing by children, < 7 years of age, should be supervised and only a pea sized amount or smear of toothpaste should be used.	Type 2,4,5
Rinsing behaviour	Discourage rinsing with large volumes of water. Encourage young children to spit out excess toothpaste.	Type 4,5
When to brush	Brush last thing at night and on one other occasion.	Type 4,5
Type of fluoride	Toothpastes containing sodium fluoride, sodium monofluorophosphate or stannous fluoride are clinically effective.	Type 1,5
Age to commence brushing	Advise parents/carers to begin brushing once the primary teeth have commenced eruption.	Type 4,5

Recommendation: Toothpastes containing sodium fluoride, sodium monofluorophosphate or a combination are clinically effective.
Evidence: (Type 1, 5)

Age to commence brushing
Several studies have reported an association between the age that toothbrushing was claimed to have commenced and caries experience (Type 4). Overall, 12% of 1.5–4.5 year olds who started to brush before the age of 1 year had some caries experience (active decay, filled teeth or teeth missing due to decay) compared with 19% who started between the ages of 1 and 2 years and 34% of those who did not start toothbrushing until after the age of 2 years.[1] Again, these data need to be treated with caution because of confounding factors.
Recommendation: Advise parents/carers to commence brushing once the primary teeth have commenced eruption.
Evidence: (Type 4,5)

PERIODONTAL DISEASE
Although plaque is the primary aetiological agent for periodontal disease it is evident that there is considerable variation in the extent and severity of tissue destruction between individuals, teeth and tooth sites.[6] The aim is to maintain a level of plaque control which ensures that the rate of tissue destruction is reduced sufficiently to ensure that most individuals maintain a comfortable and functional natural dentition for life. However, the level of plaque control required varies from individual to individual.

The oral care industry continues to try and provide the public with toothbrushes and toothpastes that improve the effectiveness of plaque control and periodontal health. The efficacy of these different products has been evaluated in numerous clinical trials the results of which have been the subject of a number of traditional reviews.[35,37]

Frequency of brushing
The effective removal of plaque every second day has been shown to prevent gingivitis[38] and resolve experimental gingivitis;[39] the less frequent removal of plaque did not prevent or reduce gingivitis. No optimum frequency has been determined but there is a consensus that twice daily brushing is consistent with maintaining good gingival health.[35,40]
Recommendation: Brush twice daily.
Evidence: (Type 5)

Brushing duration and technique
Individuals rarely brush for the length of time they say they do[41–43] and rarely exceed 60 seconds.[44,45] Most use a simple horizontal brushing action, spend little time brushing lingual areas, and fail to remove plaque effectively from the approximal surfaces of premolars and molars.[46] Traditional reviews of the literature (Type 5) have concluded that no particular method is superior to any other and it is more realistic to

modify the patient's existing method of brushing, emphasising the need to repeat the procedure on all available tooth surfaces.[35,47]
Recommendation: Modify existing method of brushing, emphasising a systematic approach to maximise plaque removal.
Evidence: (Type 5)

Manual toothbrushes
The published literature on the relative merits of different manual toothbrushes is extensive. In general (Type 5) it is accepted that toothbrushes should have the following attributes: a handle size appropriate to the user's age and dexterity, a head size appropriate to the user's mouth, a compact arrangement of soft, end rounded nylon filaments not larger than 0.009 inches in diameter and bristle patterns which enhance plaque removal in the approximal spaces and along the gum margin.[48] In an effort to improve the efficacy of plaque removal toothbrushes with filaments arranged at different heights and angles have been developed. Several randomised controlled studies (Type 2) have demonstrated that these designs were significantly more effective at removing plaque[49,50] and reducing gingivitis[52] than flat trim brushes.
Recommendation: Use a small headed brush with soft, round ended filaments, a compact, angled arrangement of long and short filaments and comfortable handle.
Evidence: (Type 2,5)

Powered toothbrushes
Most modern powered toothbrushes have a small, circular head which performs oscillating, rotating or counter-rotational movements. Timers are now being introduced into the design giving the user feedback on the duration of brushing. Numerous clinical trials have been performed comparing the efficacy of such toothbrushes with other models or manual toothbrushes. Traditional reviews[53] have generally concluded (Type 5) that powered toothbrushes are more effective in removing plaque, and in some instances reducing gingivitis, than manual toothbrushes.[3] A recent Cochrane Review[54] concluded (Type 1) that powered toothbrushes with an oscillating/rotating movement were more effective in removing plaque and reducing gingivitis than a manual toothbrush. Two studies have reported that powered toothbrushes improved compliance.[55,56] Ideally dental professionals should provide advice and instruction in the use of these devices.[57]
Recommendation: For those individuals who are unable to maintain an effective level of plaque control and periodontal health powered brushes with an oscillating/rotating action may be more effective than manual brushes.
Evidence: (Type 1,5)

Toothpaste
Since most individuals are unable to maintain an effective level of plaque control by mechanical means alone, various chemical agents have

> The profession should advise and encourage individuals to maintain an effective level of oral hygiene

been added to toothpastes to enhance the removal of plaque and thereby improve periodontal health. The most widely used agent in toothpastes is triclosan, a broad-spectrum antibacterial agent. The effectiveness of triclosan formulations has been improved by either adding a copolymer to enhance its retention in the mouth or by adding zinc citrate to provide additional antibacterial activity. These formulations have been shown in randomised controlled trials (Type 2) to provide significant reductions in plaque and significant improvements in gingival health[58,59] when compared with a fluoride toothpaste alone. In studies of 3 years duration the triclosan/copolymer formulation was reported to reduce the onset of periodontitis in adolescents[60] and the further progression of periodontitis in at- risk adults.[61]

Recommendation: Use toothpastes which contain triclosan with either copolymer or zinc citrate to improve levels of plaque control and periodontal health.

Evidence: (Type 2)

PROFESSIONAL INVOLVEMENT

The profession has a wider responsibility for preventing and controlling dental diseases than simply providing toothbrushing advice. The effectiveness of intensive professional involvement in preventive programmes has been well documented in a number of longitudinal studies. In a 4-year trial (Type 2) children, aged 7–14 years, were allocated to test and control groups.[62] During the first 2 years those in the test group received oral hygiene instruction, a professional prophylaxis and topical application of sodium monofluorophosphate every 2 weeks. During the third year this programme was repeated once a month and in the final year every 2 months. The control group brushed their teeth with a 0.32% solution of sodium fluoride once a month throughout the 4 years. Children in the test group had virtually no plaque and gingivitis and had a very small caries increment when compared with the control group. A similar programme was evaluated in adults (Type 2) over a 6-year period.[63] During the first 2 years the test group received preventive measures every 2 months and during the subsequent 4 years every 3 months. The preventive measures comprised: instruction and practice in oral

hygiene with emphasis on interdental cleaning, a professional prophylaxis and topical application of fluoride. The control group was recalled at yearly intervals and received conventional care. The preventive programme improved periodontal health and reduced the progression of periodontitis and the incidence of caries when compared with the control group. During a further 9 years the test group continued to receive the preventive programme at varying intervals depending on perceived risk.[64] Sixty-five per cent of subjects were recalled once a year, 30% twice a year and 5% at 2–4 monthly intervals. The results demonstrated that the programme effectively prevented recurrence of dental disease in all but a small number of highly susceptible individuals.

Whilst such studies clearly indicate the effectiveness of a combination of personal and professional plaque control measures in controlling dental diseases, the frequency of recall which ranged from 2 weeks to 4 months is probably unrealistic for most patients and practices.

SUMMARY

The advice that dental practitioners and hygienists give to their patients on toothbrushing should be based on the best available evidence, with due consideration being given to the individual patient's ability to achieve and maintain an acceptable level of oral health. Increasingly, systematic reviews[12,54,65] and Clinical Guidelines[66,67] are being published to support recommendations. This review indicates that much of what we advise is based on traditional reviews of the literature in which the selection of studies does not entail an appraisal of their quality. However, the number of high quality systematic reviews is increasing and will provide stronger evidence to support the advice we give and Clinical Guidelines.

Most people perceive toothbrushing as a tedious procedure which is performed primarily to provide cosmetic rather than health benefits. The increasing popularity of powered brushes and fluoride toothpastes which contain agents that also improve plaque control and periodontal health are to be welcomed. Clinician's can maximise the health benefits of this process by advising patients about frequency, choice of

Despite improvements in oral health there is still the potential for many individuals to gain greater benefit. The clinician has a clear role in providing appropriate advice to enable patients to maximise the effects of toothbrushing. Future services should recognise and support the profession in this role

Table 2 The levels of evidence for recommendations for control of periodontal disease

	Instructions	Evidence
Frequency of brushing	Twice daily	Type 5
Brushing duration and technique	Modify existing method of brushing emphasising a systematic approach.	Type 5
Manual toothbrushes	Small headed; soft, round ended filaments; compact, angled arrangement of long and short filaments; comfortable handle.	Type 2,5
Powered toothbrushes	Powered brushes may be more effective than manual brushes.	Type 1,5
Toothpaste	Toothpastes containing triclosan with either copolymer or zinc citrate provide improved levels of plaque control and periodontal health.	Type 2

toothpaste and brush, post-brush rinsing and the supervision of children.

In the UK only 62% of dentate adults recalled having been given some advice or information about toothbrushing or gum care. Patients should be given advice and encouragement to achieve and maintain an acceptable level of oral health. The advice should be tailored to the individual and reinforced at regular intervals if the desired behaviour and benefits are to be sustained.

Affiliation: Robin Davies and Roger Ellwood are employees of Colgate-Palmolive (UK) Ltd.

1. Hinds K, Gregory J R. *National Diet and Nutrition Survey; children aged 1.5 to 4.5 years. Vol 2: Report of the Dental Survey.* London: The Stationery Office, 1995.
2. Walker A, Gregory J, Bradnock G, Nunn J, White D. *National Diet and Nutrition Survey: young people aged 4 to 18 years. Vol 2: Report of the Oral Health Survey.* London: The Stationery Office, 2000.
3. Kelly M, Steele J, Nuttall N *et al. Adult Dental Health Survey: Oral Health in the United Kingdom 1998.* Walker A, Cooper I, (eds) London: The Stationery Office, 2000.
4. Clarkson J E, Worthington H V, Davies R M. Restorative treatment provided over five years for adults regularly attending general dental practice. *J Dent* 2000; **28:** 233-239.
5. Nunn J, Morris J, Pine C, Pitts N B, Bradnock G, Steele J. The conditions of teeth in the UK in 1998 and implications for the future. *Br Dent J* 2000; **189:** 639-644.
6. Morris A J, Steele J, White D A. The oral cleanliness and periodontal health of UK adults in 1998. *Br Dent J* 2001; **191:** 186-192.
7. Reisine S T, Psoter W. Socioeconomic status and selected behavioural determinants as risk factors for dental caries. *J Dent Educ* 2001; **65:** 1009-1016.
8. Sutcliffe P. Oral cleanliness and dental caries. *In* Murray J J (ed) *Prevention of oral diseases.* pp 68-77. Oxford: Oxford University Press, 1996.
9. Hotz P R. Dental plaque control and dental caries. *In* Lang N P, Attstrom R, Loe H (eds) *Proceedings of the European Workshop on Mechanical Plaque Control.* pp 35-49. Chicago: Quintessence, 1998.
10. Koch G, Lindhe J. The state of the gingivae and caries increment in school children during and after withdrawal of various prophylactic measures. *In* McHugh W D (ed) *Dental Plaque.* pp 271-281. Edinburgh: Livingstone, 1970.
11. Bratthall D, Hansel Peterson G, Sundberg H. Reasons for the caries decline: what do the experts believe? *Euro J Oral Sci* 1996; **104:** 416-422.
12. Marinho V C C, Higgins J P T, Sheiham A, Logan S. Fluoride toothpastes for preventing dental caries in children and adolescents (Cochrane Review). *In: The Cochrane Library,* Issue 1. 2003. Oxford: Update Software.
13. Chesters R K, Huntington E, Burchell C K, Stephen K. W. Effect of oral care habits on caries in adolescents. *Caries Res* 1992; **26:** 299-304.
14. Chestnutt I G, Schafer K, Jacobson A P M, Stephen K W. The influence of toothbrushing frequency and post-brushing rinsing on caries experience in a caries clinical trial. *Community Dent Oral Epidemiol* 1998; **26:** 406-411.
15. *The Scientific Basis of Dental Health Education: A Policy Document* (revised fourth edition). Health Development Agency 2001.
16. Clarkson J E, Ellwood R P, Chandler R E. A comprehensive summary of fluoride dentifrice caries clinical trials. *Am J Dent* 1993; **6:** (Spec Iss) S59-S106.
17. Stephen K W, Creanor S L, Russell J I *et al.* A 3 year oral health dose response study of sodium monofluorophosphate dentifrices with and without zinc citrate: anticaries results. *Community Dent Oral Epidemiol* 1988; **16:** 321-325.
18. Ammari A B, Bloch-Zupan A, Ashley P F. Systematic review of studies comparing the anti-caries activity of children's toothpaste containing 600 ppm of fluoride or less with high fluoride toothpastes of 1,000 ppm or above. *Caries Res* 2003; **37:** 85-92.
19. Winter G B, Holt R D, Williams B F. Clinical trial of a low fluoride toothpaste for young children. *Int Dent J* 1989; **39:** 227-235.
20. Davies G M, Worthington H V, Ellwood R P *et al.* A randomised controlled trial of the effectiveness of providing free toothpaste from the age of 12 months on reducing caries in 56-year old children. *Community Dental Health* 2002; **19:** 131-136.
21. Marks R G, D'Agostino R, Moorhead J E *et al.* A fluoride dose response evaluation in an anti-caries clinical trial. *J Dent Res* 1992; **71:** 1286-1291
22. Biesbrock A R, Gerlach R W, Bollmer B W, Faller R V, Jacobs S A, Bartizek R D. Relative anti-caries efficacy of 1100, 1700, 2200, and 2800 ppm fluoride ion in a sodium fluoride dentifrice over 1 year. *Community Dent Oral Epidemiol* 2001; **29:** 382-389.
23. Hausen H. Caries prediction-state of the art. *Community Dent Oral Epidemiol* 1997; **25:** 87-96.
24. Disney J A, Graves R C, Stamm J W, Bohannon H M, Abernathy J R, Zack D D, The University of North Carolina Caries Risk Assessment study: further developments in caries risk prediction. *Community Dent Oral Epidemiol* 1992; **20:** 64-75.
25. O'Mullane D M, Kavanagh D, Ellwood R P *et al.* A three year clinical trial of a combination of trimetaphosphate and sodium fluoride in silica toothpastes. *J Dent Res* 1997; **76:** 1776-1778.
26. Duckworth R M, Morgan S N. Oral fluoride retention after use of fluoride dentifrices. *Caries Res* 1991; **25:** 123-129.
27. Sjogren K, Birkhed D. Factors related to fluoride retention after toothbrushing and possible connection to caries activity. *Caries Res* 1993; **27:** 474-477.
28. Duckworth R M, Morgan S N, Murray A M. Fluoride in saliva and plaque following use of dentifrices containing sodium monofluorophosphate. *J Dent Res* 1989; **68:** 130-133.
29. Bentley E M. Ellwood R P, Davies R M. Fluoride ingestion from toothpaste by young children. *Br Dent J* 1999; **186:** 460-462.
30. Levy S M. Review of fluoride exposures and ingestion. *Community Dent Oral Epidemiol* 1994; **22:** 173-180.
31. British Society of Paediatric Dentistry: A policy document on fluoride dietary supplements and fluoride toothpastes for children. *Int J Paed Dent* 1996; **6:** 139-142.
32. Duckworth R M, Moore S S. Salivary fluoride concentrations after overnight use of toothpastes. *Caries Res* 2001; **35:** 285.
33. Johnson M F. Comparative efficacy of NaF and SMFP dentifrices in caries prevention: a meta-analytic overview. *Caries Res* 1993; **27:** 328-336.
34. Holloway P J, Worthington H V. Sodium fluoride or sodium monofluorophosphate? A critical review of a meta-analysis on their relative effectiveness in dentifrices. *Am J Dent* 1993; **6:** (Spec Iss) S55-S58.
35. Jepsen S. The role of manual toothbrushes in effective plaque control: Advantages and limitations. *In* Lang NP, Attstrom R, Loe H. (eds) *Proceedings of the European Workshop on Mechanical Plaque Removal.* pp 121-137. Chicago: Quintessence, 1998.
36. van der Weijden G A, Timmerman M F, Danser M M, van der Velden U. The role of electric toothbrushes: Advantages and Limitations. *In* Lang N P, Attstrom R, Loe H (eds) *Proceedings of the European Workshop on Mechanical Plaque Control.* pp 138-155. Chicago: Quintessence, 1998.
37. Adriaens P A, Gjermo P. Anti-plaque and anti-gingivitis efficacy of toothpastes. *In* Lang N P, Karring T, Lindhe J. (eds) *Proceedings of the 2nd European Workshop on Periodontology. Chemicals in periodontics.* pp 204-220. Chicago: Quintessence, 1997.
38. Lang N P, Cumming B R, Loe H. Toothbrushing frequency as it relates to plaque development and gingival health. *J Periodont* 1973; **44:** 396-405.
39. Bosman C W, Powell R N. The reversal of localized experimental gingivitis. *J Clin Periodontol* 1977; **4:** 161-172.
40. Addy M, Adriens P. Consensus report of Group A. Epidmiology and etiology of periodontal diseases and the role of plaque control in dental caries. *In* Lang N P, Attstrom R, Loe H (eds) *Proceedings of the European Workshop on Mechanical Plaque Control.* pp 98-101. Chicago: Quintessence, 1998.
41. Macgregor I D M, Rugg-Gunn A J. A survey of toothbrushing duration in 85 uninstructed English school children. *Community Dent Oral Epidemiol* 1979; **7:** 297-298.
42. Cancro L P, Fischman S L. The expected effect on oral health of dental plaque control through mechanical removal. *Periodontol* 2000 1995; **8:** 60-74.
43. Saxer U P, Emling R C, Yankel S L. Actual vs estimated tooth brushing time and tooth paste used. *Caries Res* 1983; **17:** 179-180.
44. Rugg-Gunn A J, MacGregor I D M. A survey of toothbrushing

behaviour in children and young adults. *J Perio Res* 1978; **113:** 382-388.

45. Yankell S L. Toothbrushing and toothbrushing techniques. *In* Harris N O, Christen A G. (eds) *Primary preventive dentistry.* 3rd ed. Norwalk C T: Appleton and Lange, 1991.

46. Hawkins R J, Zanetti D L, Main P A *et al.* Toothbrushing competency among high-risk grade one students: an evaluation of two methods of dental health education. *J Public Health Dent* 2001; **61:** 197-202.

47. Egelberg J. *Oral Hygiene Methods, The Scientific Way, Synopsis of Clinical Studies.* p13 Malmo: OdontoScience, 1999.

48. Egelberg J, Claffey N. Role of mechanical dental plaque removal in prevention and therapy of caries and periodontal diseases. *In* Lang N P, Attstrom,R, Loe, H (eds) *Proceedings of the European Workshop on Mechanical Plaque Control.* pp 169-172. Chicago: Quintessence, 1998.

49. Balanyk T E, Sharma N C, Galustians J. A clinical study of comparative plaque removal performance of two manual toothbrushes. *J Clin Dent* 1993; **4:** (Suppl D) D8-D12.

50. Sharma N C, Rustogi K N, McCool J J *et al.* Comparative plaque removal efficacy of three toothbrushes in two independent clinical studies. *J Clin Dent* 1992; **3:** (Suppl C) C13-C28.

51. Cronin M J, Dembling W Z, Low M L, Jacobs D M, Weber D A. A comparative clinical investigation of a novel toothbrush designed to enhance plaque removal efficacy. *Am J Dent* 2000; **13:** (Spec Iss) 21A-26A.

52. Sharma N C, Galustians J, McCool J J, Rustogi K N, Volpe A R. The clinical effects on plaque and gingivitis over 3 months use of four complex design manual toothbrushes. *J Clin Dent* 1994; **5:** 114-118.

53. Heasman P A, McCracken G I. Powered toothbrushes: a review of clinical trials. *J Clin Periodontol* 1999; **26:** 407-420.

54. Heanue M, Deacon S A, Deery C *et al.* Manual versus powered toothbrushing for oral health. (Cochrane Review). In: *The Cochrane Library, Issue 1.* 2003. Oxford. Software Update.

55. Hellstadius K, Asman B, Gustafsson A. Improved maintenance of plaque control by electrical toothbrushing in periodontitis patients with low compliance. *J Clin Periodontol* 1993; **20:** 235-237.

56. Stalnacke K, Soderfelt B, Sjodin B. Compliance in use of electric toothbrushes. *Acta Odont Scand* 1995; **53:** 17-19.

57. Renton-Harper P, Addy M, Newcombe R G. Plaque removal with the uninstructed use of electric toothbrushes; comparison with a manual brush and toothpaste slurry. *J Clin Periodontol* 2001; **28:** 325-330.

58. Svatun B, Saxton C A, Rolla G, van der Ouderaa F G H. A 1-year study on the efficacy of a dentifrice containing zinc citrate and triclosan to maintain gingival health. *Scand J Dent Res* 1989; **97:** 242-246.

59. Volpe A R, Petrone M E, DeVizio W, Davies R M, Proskin H M. A review of plaque, gingivitis, calculus and caries clinical efficacy studies with a fluoride dentifrice containing triclosan and PVM /MA copolymer. *J Clin Dent* 1996; **7** (Suppl): S1-S14.

60. Ellwood R P, Worthington H.V, Blinkhorn A S B, Volpe A R, Davies R M. Effect of a triclosan/copolymer dentifrice on the incidence of periodontal attachment loss in adolescents. *J Clin Periodontol* 1998; **25:** 363-367.

61. Rosling B, Wannfors B, Volpe A R, Furuichi Y, Ramberg P, Lindhe J. The use of a triclosan/copolymer dentifrice may retard the progression of periodontitis. *J Clin Periodontol* 1997; **24:** 873-88.

62. Axelsson P, Lindhe J. The effect of a plaque control program on gingivitis and dental caries in schoolchildren. *J Dent Res* 1977; **56** (Spec Iss C): C142-C148.

63. Axelsson P, Lindhe J. Effect of controlled oral hygiene procedures on caries and periodontal disease in adults. Results after 6 years. *J Clin Periodontol* 1981; **8:** 239-248.

64. Axelsson P, Lindhe J, Nystrom B. On the prevention of caries and periodontal disease. Results of a 15-year longitudinal study. *J Clin Periodontol* 1991; **18:** 182-189.

65. NIH Consensus Development Conference on Diagnosis and Management of Dental Caries throughout life. *J Dent Educ* 2001; **65:** 935-1179.

66. *National Clinical Guidelines 1997.* London: The Royal College of Surgeons of England.

67. *Health Evidence Bulletins Wales, Oral Health.* Cardiff. Welsh Office.1998.

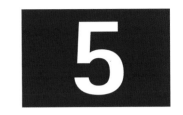
IN BRIEF

- A preventive strategy at the planning stage describing patient selection, surgical technique, prosthetic design and loading
- A preventive strategy for the maintenance period describing recall examination and diagnosis and therapy
- The level of evidence currently available to support these strategies

Prevention. Part 5: Preventive strategies for patients requiring osseointegrated oral implant treatment

P. Coulthard[1], M. Esposito[2], M. Slater[3] and H. V. Worthington[4]; Series Editor E. J. Kay[5]

Prevention for patients requiring rehabilitation with oral implants is about preventing implant failure and biomechanical complications. This paper describes preventative strategies for the planning stage for implant treatment and the later maintenance period and indicates the level of scientific evidence supporting these strategies.

PREVENTION

1. Smoking cessation advice
2. Dietary advice
3. Prevention of tooth wear
4. Toothbrushing advice
5. **Patients requiring osseointegrated oral implant treatment**
6. Older dentate patient
7. Professionally applied topical fluorides for caries prevention
8. Pit and fissure sealants in preventing caries in the permanent dentition of children

[1]Senior Lecturer and Honorary Consultant, Head of Oral and Maxillofacial Surgery, University Dental Hospital of Manchester; [2]Assistant Researcher, Department of Biomaterials and Department of Prosthetic Dentistry/Dental Material Sciences, The Sahlgrenska Academy at Göteborg University, Göteborg, Sweden; [3]Principal Tutor, Head of Oral Health Sciences, University Dental Hospital of Manchester; [4]Co-ordinating Editor, Cochrane Oral Health Group, University Dental Hospital of Manchester [5]Professor of Dental Health Services Research, University of Manchester Dental Hospital and School, Higher Cambridge Street, Manchester M15 6FH
Correspondence to: Dr Paul Coulthard, Oral and Maxillofacial Surgery, University Dental Hospital of Manchester, Higher Cambridge Street,. Manchester M15 6FH
Email: paul.coulthard@man.ac.uk

Missing teeth and supporting oral tissues have traditionally been replaced with dentures or bridges permitting the restoration of masticatory, phonetic function, and aesthetics. Dental implants now offer an alternative for tooth replacement. Inserted into the mandible or maxilla, these implants are retained because of the intimacy of bone growth onto their surface so that they can support a dental prosthesis. Osseointegration is the word used to describe the healing of bone around implants so that there is direct anchorage of the implant that is then maintained during functional loading without the growth of fibrous tissue at the bone-implant interface.[1]

Prevention for patients requiring rehabilitation with oral implants is about preventing implant failure. Biological failure occurs when osseointegration is not established or is not maintained. When not established in the first place, implant failure is described as 'early failure' and will be observed before or at abutment connection. When osseointegration does occur but then is lost, the implant failure is described as a 'late failure' as this is observed at any time after abutment connection. When an implant is not osseointegrated, a peri-implant radiolucency is observed radiographically and the implant is clinically mobile. It is obviously important to prevent implant failure through adequate planning to facilitate establishment of osseointegration and then to preserve the long-term maintenance of osseointegration. This paper describes preventive strategies for the planning stage (Table 1) for implant treatment and the later maintenance period (Table 2) and indicates the level of scientific evidence supporting these strategies.

Table 1 Factors in preventive strategy at planning stage

Patient selection

- General health
- Smoking
- Bone quality and other anatomical factors
- Oral hygiene
- History of radiotherapy

Surgical technique

- Surgical trauma
- Number of implants
- Type of implant
- Microbial contamination
- Antibiotic usage

Loading

Prosthetic design

Table 2 Factors in preventive strategy for the maintenance period

Recall examination and diagnosis

- Examination of the prosthesis
- Examination of the implants

Therapy

- Patient administered hygiene procedures
- Mechanical debridement by the professional
- Pharmacological therapy
- Surgical procedures

PREVENTIVE STRATEGY AT THE PLANNING STAGE

Patient Selection

General Health
It seems likely that systemic conditions that interfere with wound healing also interfere with implant osseointegration, although there are actually few studies looking specifically at particular medical conditions. Patients with systemic diseases such as diabetes mellitus, or those taking systemic steroid therapy or other immunosuppressive medication are known to have impaired wound healing and these patients are often thought to also have an increased rate of implant failure. Many of the published reports specifically investigating diabetes include too few patients to offer conclusive results.[2,3] A study analysing data from the Department of Veteran Affairs Dental Implant Registry in the USA observed an association between the medical history in general of a patient and implant failure.[4] This was then reported by a conference seeking consensus on variables predictive of implant failure (Perio Consensus Report 1996).[5] However, regarding diabetes, this publication reported no greater implant failure rate in patients with well-controlled diabetes mellitus than observed in the general population.

Smoking
Several observational studies have described a relationship between smoking and increased implant failure but the strength of this relationship varies between studies. One study has shown only a 0.6 mm mean difference in bone levels between smoking and non-smoking groups over a 10-year period, which is of little clinical significance.[6] More recently a study reported smokers to have a one and a half times the 6% failure rate observed in patients of the group who had never smoked.[7] Implants in the maxilla had almost two times the risk of failure in smokers than non-smokers. The authors of this study suggested that the increased failure rate was caused by the exposure of the peri-implant tissues to tobacco smoke. Other researchers have also implicated altered peri-implant tissue conditions.[8-10] Generally there is a consensus that smokers have about twice the number of failed implants compared with non-smokers, although well-designed trials are lacking.

Bone quality and other anatomical factors
Implant success is related to the quality of the bone into which the implant is inserted and therefore this factor should be taken into account when planning the placement site of the implants. Site seems to be an important factor irrespective of whether the implants are loaded or not.[11-13] Higher failure rates have been reported for implants placed in maxillary bone compared with mandibular bone and also in the posterior segments of both jaws. Posterior sites

may also restrict the bone volume available for placement of large implants because of vital structures such as the inferior alveolar nerve or maxillary sinus.[14] A reduced success rate has also been described when bone grafting is undertaken to facilitate implant placement at sites of inadequate volume.[16] Bone quality seems to relate primarily to bone density and the denser the bone, the fewer the failures, with the exception of extremely dense bone. The presence of dense bone may favour early implant stability, which is one of the prerequisites for predictable osseointegration. Interestingly, it has been shown in a laboratory model that the maximum stresses and strains are concentrated about the crestal cortical bone rather than the cancellous bone and that from a biomechanical point of view, implants may be almost completely supported by the cortical bone, when present.[15]

Oral hygiene
The patient should have demonstrated the ability to maintain proper hygiene before proceeding with implant treatment as a cause-effect relationship between bacterial plaque accumulation and the development of inflammatory changes in the soft tissues surrounding oral implants has been shown.[17] However, no relationship between previous periodontal disease and implant failure has been established yet.[18-20]

Several studies have indicated that remaining teeth might act as a reservoir for the colonization of the subgingival area around implants.[21,22] This suggested that there may be an association between susceptibility for periodontitis and susceptibility for peri-implantitis, especially in partially edentulous patients. However, a recent study has failed to find any relationship between ongoing periodontitis around teeth and bone loss around implants inserted in the same jaw. Patients were included in this study with either a history of stabilised or progressive periodontitis and patients had no more marginal bone loss than patients with a healthy periodontium when measured radiographically and clinically.[23]

Keratinised mucosa
It has been suggested that an adequate band of keratinised mucosa about an implant is necessary for its success[24,25] but it has not been possible to demonstrate this scientifically[26] and the consensus view now is that there is no correlation between the width of keratinised mucosa and implant failure.[5] However, it may be that the presence of keratinised tissue facilitates the patients' hygiene procedures but in many patients these may be adequate without keratinised tissue.[11] Similarly, an adequate sulcus is required for plaque control and to avoid tissue tension involving the peri-implant soft tissues.

Radiotherapy
Individual observational studies of implant failure rates in irradiated and non-irradiated patients have been compared. This has shown

Smoking

Generally there is a consensus that smokers have about twice the number of failed implants compared with non-smokers, although well-designed trials are lacking

that failure rates in the mandibles of irradiated patients are slightly higher than those of non-irradiated patients but that irradiated maxillas show a much higher failure rate than irradiated mandibles.[27] The failure rate was also shown to be dose dependent with an increased failure rate at higher radiation doses.

As fibrosis and loss of micro-vascularity begins about 6 months after irradiation and then progressively worsens,[28] implant treatment should probably be undertaken early. Whilst there is much support for the use of hyperbaric oxygen therapy for these patients from observational studies, there is a dearth of high-level evidence from randomised controlled trials (RCTs) evidence supporting or rejecting its benefits.[29]

Genetic factors
Differences in genetic makeup that reflect differences in healing or other factors may relate to implant success, but at present there is still no available information.

Surgical technique

Surgical trauma
Prevention of failure should also take into account the surgery. This should be undertaken as atraumatically as possible and implants should be placed using drills at appropriate speed and with adequate irrigation to prevent bone heating. If the temperature is permitted to rise to over 47°C for 1 minute, then this may cause a zone of necrotic bone surrounding the inserted implant and it is thought that this may be clinically significant.[30,31]

Number of implants
An adequate number of correctly positioned implants should be planned as part of the loading consideration. Excess loading may lead to biological failure, that is, loss of osseointegration, but also to mechanical failure of the implants or retained prosthesis. There is some evidence from a few studies to show that the number of implants supporting a fixed prosthesis may be important for treatment success.[6,32] Three or more implants seems to be more successful than two implants for the rehabilitation of partially dentate patients.

Implant type
Implant surface characteristics such as roughness and type of coating may influence the failure pattern and numerous surface modifications have been developed to enhance clinical performance. A recent systematic review found that there were very few studies comparing different implant types and no evidence that any of the implant systems evaluated was superior to the another.[33] Those studies included investigated Astra, Branemark, IMZ, ITI, Steri-Oss and Southern implant systems. However, these findings were based on a few RCTs all having short follow-up periods and few study patients.

Microbial contamination
A high standard of cross-infection control should be adopted for implant surgery as a correlation has been observed between increasing numbers of implants placed in a patient and increased failure rate.[34] The authors of this study suggested that this could have been due to the longer operating time and consequent larger wound contamination. A larger failure rate has also been reported in patients with high plaque scores likely as a result of bacterial contamination at the time of implant placement.[35] It is also known that biomaterial infections are extremely resistant to host defence mechanisms and antibiotic therapy.[36] Microorganisms preferentially adhere to implant surfaces and form a biofilm to protect themselves from the host.[37] The shape of the implant therefore may also have a bearing on infection rate. Hollow implants used in orthopaedic surgery (intramedullary nails) have been found to have an infection rate almost two times that of solid nails but this was from an animal study rather than a clinical trial.[38] Similarly, implants with a porous surface have been reported to have more early infections than dense implant.[39]

Antibiotic usage
It is common practice to use prophylactic antibiotics or a course of antibiotics after implant placement to increase the success although this practice remains controversial. There is some evidence from observational studies that preoperative antibiotics reduce the early failure rate [40] although no randomised controlled trial has been carried out yet. Chlorhexidine mouthrinse used pre-operatively is also associated with a reduced complication rate.[41]

Loading
Excessive loading in relation to bone quality is another cause of implant failure.[11,23] It has been suggested that implants should not be loaded during a healing phase of 3–4 months in the mandible and 6–8 months in the maxilla if osseointegration is to occur.[1] Some studies comparing immediately loaded and conventionally loaded Branemark mandibular implants showed an overall seven times higher early failure rate for those immediately loaded.[42,43] Experimental evidence has indicated that early loading causes micromovement of the implant and differentiation of cells into fibroblasts resulting in fibrous encapsulation rather than osseointegration.[44] Alternatively, other laboratory experiments have shown that daily low frequency micromotion may stimulate bone growth.[45] The precise level of micromotion that can be tolerated clinically without significantly inhibiting bone formation is unknown.

Recently, immediate and early loaded implants are being used particularly in the mandible.[46] It is likely that the bone quality is of major importance for success in this situation. Some authors are also advocating implant surface modifications as a means of facilitating the

Implant type

A recent systematic review found that there were very few studies comparing different implant types and no evidence that any of the implant systems evaluated was superior to the another earlier loading of implants.[47] There are an inadequate number of good quality randomised controlled trials comparing immediate versus conventionally loaded implants[48] and also the related question of whether to close over soft tissues during healing (two-stage surgery) or to leave exposed (one stage surgery) to provide clear evidence for practice.[33]

Whilst there is little clinical evidence that bruxism or clenching parafunctions are associated with increased implant failure, there seems to be general consensus that excessive loading may induce bone loss. It is actually difficult to obtain good evidence as it is difficult to clinically quantify the magnitude and direction of bite forces applied by a patient in relation to the bone quality and control groups.[49]

Prosthetic design

The planned type of prosthesis, crown, fixed bridge or overdenture, has implications for maintenance by the patient. The implant plan should aim to achieve an emergence profile that enables easy cleaning. The suprastructure should be designed so that the patient can maintain proper oral hygiene. If the reconstruction is overcontoured, especially interproximally, this will prevent the achievement of optimal oral hygiene.[50]

It has been suggested that cantilever length influences stress distribution, particularly on distal implants,[51] but only a few studies have investigated this. One study reported that cantilevers longer than 15 mm had to be remade more often than shorter cantilevers.[52]

PREVENTIVE STRATEGY FOR THE MAINTENANCE PERIOD

The aim after completion of implant and restoration is to prevent implant failure by offering the patient a programme designed for his or her individual needs

Examination and diagnosis

It is generally recommended that patients should be reviewed regularly. The recall interval may be 6 months but will vary according to the patient's individual needs. There are no cost benefit analyses studies relating to this view. The examination should focus on the prosthesis, the implants and the peri-implant tissues.

Examination of the prosthesis

This should include noting the retention and stability, any abutment or screw loosening or loss of cement. The occlusion should be examined.

Examination of the implants:

• Mobility

Pain or sensitivity when eating or when the abutment screw is tightened may be an early indication of osseointegration failure. However, it is important to bear in mind that failed implants can be completely asymptomatic. Any indication of mobility indicates a failed implant

as a result of loss of osseointegration and is occasionally present when radiographic bone changes are not distinct. For research purposes, the prosthesis may need to be removed but this would be unreasonable in normal clinical practice at review appointments and mobility testing cannot be carried out if implants are supporting a cemented prosthesis. Radiographic examination, whilst not as accurate a test for implant failure as mobility, provides a good indication and avoids having to remove a fixed prosthesis.

The Periotest electronic device provides an objective measure of mobility although it does not provide an indication of implant failure any earlier than indicated by radiographic changes.[53] Several factors have an influence on Periotest values including, the length of the implant and abutment, whether the implant is in mandibular or maxillary bone, and bone density.

It has been proposed that at abutment connection, a 10 N cm reverse torque could be applied to the implant to check for mobility but this may risk damaging a weak immature bone/implant interface and is therefore not recommended.[54] Other non-invasive evaluation methods are now available but the correlation between their measures and osseointegration are not clear.[55,56] Simply to know whether an implant is mobile or not may be more clinically relevant.

• Radiographs

Periapical radiographs should be taken to show the bone level about implants. These should be taken in a standardised way so that they are reproducible and avoid distortion. Dental panoramic radiographs are of less use than periapical radiographs, particularly for research, in monitoring bone stability about implants because of the inferior image resolution and the inability to modify the angulation of the x-ray beam.[57] A periapical radiograph should be first taken soon after abutment connection to provide a baseline measure of bone level for comparing subsequent follow-up radiographs taken to monitor any progressive marginal bone loss or 'saucerization'.[58] This bone loss may result from peri-implantitis or overloading of the implant. Regular radiographs at determined follow-up periods may not be necessary but rather should be taken to clarify some question prompted by the clinical examination.

The implant would not initially be mobile with this type of bone loss as there remains a large area of bone/implant interface osseointegration. Alternatively, a thin radiolucent peri-implant margin may be observed surrounding the entire implant, suggesting absence of osseointegration and a loss of stability.[59] When excessive marginal bone loss or a radiolucent peri-implant margin is observed then the implant mobility should be checked and this may require removal of a bridge.

Less than 1.5 mm of marginal bone loss during the first year of loading, and thereafter less

Radiographs

A periapical radiograph should be first taken soon after abutment connection to provide a baseline measure of bone level for comparing subsequent follow-up radiographs taken to monitor any progressive marginal bone loss or 'saucerization'

than 0.02 mm each year, has been defined as success[60] although some authors have doubted whether a firm limit for an acceptable annual bone loss can be established.[61] It is not technically possible to observe radiographic changes of 0.1 mm but threaded implants permit reference by way of the threads for serial radiographs. Another shortcoming is that only interproximal aspects of an implant can be observed.

• *Peri-implant tissues*

The attachment between an implant and the surrounding tissues is quite different from that between a tooth and the surrounding tissues, primarily because there is no periodontal ligament. Nevertheless, if an implant is biocompatible, one may expect the usual wound healing principles to establish healthy peri-implant tissues. One of the key factors for the long-term success of oral implants is the maintenance of healthy tissues around them.[62]

A cause-effect relationship between bacterial plaque accumulation and the development of inflammatory changes in the soft tissues surrounding oral implants has been shown.[17] Peri-implant mucositis is the term used to describe the reversible inflammatory changes in the tissues around an implant.[65] If this condition is left untreated, it may lead to the progressive destruction of the tissues supporting an implant (peri-implantitis) and ultimately to its failure.[63] The majority of the evidence for this association comes from microbiological observations based on observational studies. These demonstrate the presence of suspected periodontal pathogens in peri-implantitis situations or the presence of the usual microorganisms associated with health in the clinically healthy situation.[65,66] For maintaining healthy tissues around oral implants it is important to institute an effective preventive regimen and, when a pathological condition of the tissues around implants has been diagnosed, then a therapeutic intervention should be initiated as soon as possible.[67] Peri-implant inflammation is successfully treated by effective oral hygiene and plaque control as with inflammation around natural teeth. Different maintenance regimens and treatment strategies for peri-implantitis (failing implants) have been suggested, however it is unclear which are the most effective.[62,67–69]

It is not clear how reliable the various periodontal parameters are for identifying peri-implant pathology.

Bleeding on probing (BOP) is the periodontal parameter used to evaluate the presence of an inflammatory process at the base of a periodontal pocket. The presence of bleeding is noted on probing in the pocket until a slight resistance is met using gentle force. Standardised probes which produce forces of 0.25 N are available. The absence of BOP is a reliable indicator for periodontal stability[70] but the use of this measure for peri-implant tissues is not necessarily as helpful and insufficient data are currently available.

The sulcus bleeding index (SBI), is the bleeding tendency of the alveolar mucosa surrounding the implant abutment observed by running a periodontal probe along the abutment circumference 1 mm into the mucosal pocket and parallel to the margin of the soft tissues. This parameter distinguishes between healthy and inflamed tissues but may not be able to identify failing implants.[11]

Pocket probing depth (PPD), is the linear distance from the free mucosal margin to the base of the pocket. The base of the pocket is defined as the apical termination of the junctional epithelium when used for teeth but for implants there is no periodontal attachment to stop the tip of the probe. A deep pocket is a protective habitat for putative pathogens which may lead to peri-implant pathology.[71] A recent report suggested that probing measurements around osseointegrated oral implants and teeth were different. Even mild marginal inflammation was associated with deeper probe penetration around implants in comparison to teeth.[72] Pocket probing depth may not provide as accurate an indication of disease as bone level measurements on intraoral radiographs,[11] but it could still be useful in practice.

Other signs of infection such as hyperplastic tissues, suppuration, swelling, or colour change may also provide an indication that therapy is indicated. Mucosal recession exposing threads or a rough implant surface might reduce the ability of the patient to maintain the implant clean from plaque in addition to causing an aesthetic problem.

Therapy

Patient administered hygiene procedures

The patient should be instructed in brushing using soft brushes and interproximal brushes and flossing with appropriate designs of floss such as superfloss for mechanical plaque removal.[73] Adjunctive twice-daily antimicrobial mouthrinsing with an agent such as chlorhexidine has been recommended for patients with physical impairment.[73–75] Powered toothbrushes have also been recommended.[76,77] Recently a Cochrane Systematic review examined the effectivness of different maintenance therapies for patients with oral implants.[62] This review indicated that there was little available evidence for the effectiveness of interventions for maintaining healthy tissues around dental implants. However, Listerine mouthwash, 20 ml used twice a day for 30 seconds, as adjunct to routine oral hygiene was found to be effective in reducing plaque formation and improving health around implants. There was no evidence that the use of powered or sonic toothbrushes was superior to manual tooth brushing.

Mechanical debridement by the professional

Given the association between plaque and the development of pathology of the tissues about implants, it would be reasonable to arrange the following regimen, although no cost benefit

Therapy

When a pathological condition of the tissues around implants has been diagnosed, then a therapeutic intervention should be initiated as soon as possible

Scaling

Scaling with hard plastic or titanium instruments is recommended to avoid scratching and roughening the titanium implant abutment surface

analyses have been carried out. An appropriately trained professional should provide intensive motivational hygiene instruction for the patient about 1 week after abutment surgery.

After restoration this should be repeated. Remotivation and patient instruction in oral hygiene should be carried out every 6 months or at an appropriate time period for the individual patient.

Professional removal of plaque and calculus from the implant-abutment surface should be undertaken when needed. Scaling with hard plastic or titanium instruments is recommended to avoid scratching and roughening the titanium implant abutment surface that may increase the chance of bacterial colonization,[78] although all of the evidence for colonisation is derived from *in vitro* studies and no clinical trials have validated this hypothesis. Plastic scalers are also recommended to avoid galvanic corrosion and contamination of metallic implants although there is no evidence to support this.[79,80] Plastic tips for ultrasonic devices are also recommended. A rubber cup and fine abrasive polishing paste (fluor of pumice, Nupro Fine, tin oxide) might be helpful.[81]

Pharmacological therapy
Systemic antibiotics are frequently used in clinical practice as an adjunct to surgical intervention for the treatment of peri-implantitis although the evidence for their efficacy has not been clearly demonstrated.[82] Subgingival irrigation with antimicrobial agents has also been advocated for the prevention of peri-implantitis.[82] Phosphoric acid gel application has also been recommended,[81] although a recent Cochrane review on maintenance for implant patients did not find any evidence that phosphoric etching gel (monthly 35% for one minute) offered any clinical advantage over mechanical debridement.[62]

Surgical procedures
Surgical procedures have been recommended for the management of peri-implantitis.[67] In particular, open flap debridement to facilitate smoothing of the implant surface and removing unsupported implant threads that protect bacterial plaque. The implant surface may also be 'decontaminated' using various chemical agents[83] or laser energy,[84] but there is no evidence that either is necessary or effective. Once the surface has been rendered 'bacterial free', further surgery to alter the local anatomy may be necessary to enable easy plaque removal.[85]

DISCUSSION AND CONCLUSIONS

Early implant failure is most commonly attributed to excessive surgical trauma together with inadequate healing because of host compromise, premature loading and infection. The most important causes of late failure are likely to be peri-implantitis and overload together with host factors.[11,27] The common observation that failures tend to be concentrated in particular individual patients suggests that certain factors are important in determining implant success. Even though several factors have been highlighted as associated with a higher failure rate this may not preclude the patient from proceeding with implant treatment. This particularly applies to the patient selection factors. The most appropriate clinical option for tooth replacement for a patient who smokes or who has undergone radiotherapy may be implant treatment but the clinician should advise the patient as to the likely reduced success rate.

It is important to know which therapy is most effective to manage a patient and consequently the importance of evidence-based dentistry is becoming increasingly recognised. There is a general consensus that randomised controlled clinical trials (RCTs) are preferred to answer questions of therapy effectiveness, and systematic reviews can evaluate the quality of RCTs and combine their results to reach more reliable conclusions.[86] A randomised controlled trial is not however always feasible. Patients cannot be randomised to smoking, diabetes, or radiotherapy groups, for example, and so the evidence must sometimes be based on good observational studies. Systematic reviews have a clearly formulated hypothesis employing systematic methods to identify, select and critically appraise relevant research. Data from original trials are collected, analysed and if possible summarised to provide a more precise estimate of the intervention effects than available from individual trials. Unfortunately there are few RCTs as yet available investigating any management alternatives for oral implant rehabilitation.[87] Recently a Cochrane Systematic review examined the effectiveness of different maintenance therapies for patients with oral implants.[62] This review indicated that there was little available evidence for the effectiveness of interventions for maintaining healthy tissues around dental implants and the relatively few findings that were presented were based on short follow-up periods (the longest was 5 months) and there is no reliable evidence for long-term maintenance. Therefore many of the standard maintenance therapies used are not based on reliable scientific evidence. These therapies may be effective, but their efficacy needs to be demonstrated in trials and their relative cost should also be investigated.

1. Branemark P I, Hansson B O, Adell R, Breine U, Lindstrom J, Hallen O, Ohman A. Osseointegrated implants in the treatment of the edentulous jaw. Experience from a 10-year period. *Scand J Plastic Reconstructive Surg* 1977; **16**: 1-132.
2. Smith R A, Berger R, Dodson T B. Risk factors associated with dental implants in healthy and medically compromised patients. *Int J Oral Maxillofac Implants* 1992; **7**: 367-372.
3. Mericske-Stern R, Zarb G A. Overdentures: An alternative implant methodology for edentulous patients. *Int J Prosthodont* 1993; **6**: 203-208.
4. Weyant R. Characteristics associated with the loss and peri-implants tissue health of endosseous dental implants. *Int J Oral Maxillofac Implants* 1994; **9**: 95-102.
5. Proceedings of the 1996 World Workshop in Periodontics. Consensus report. Implant therapy II. *Ann Periodont* 1996; **1**: 816-820.
6. Lindquist L W, Carlsson G E, Jemt T. A prospective 15-year follow-up study of mandibular fixed prostheses supported

by osseointegrated implants. Clinical results and marginal bone loss. *Clin Oral Implants Res* 1996; **7:** 329-336.

7. Lambert P M, Morris H F, Ochi S. The influence of smoking on 3-year clinical success on osseointegrated dental implants. *Ann Periodontol* 2000; **5:** 79-89.

8. Bain C A. Smoking and implant failure-benefits of a smoking cessation protocol. *Int J Oral Maxillofac Implants* 1996; **11:** 756-759.

9. Haas R, Halmbock W, Mailath G, Watzec G. The relationship of smoking on peri-implant tissue: a retrospective study. *J Prosthet Dent* 1996; **76:** 592-596.

10. Lemons J E, Laskin D M, Roberts W E, Tarnow D P, Shipman C J, Paczkowski C, Lorey RE, English C. Changes in patient screening for a clinical study of dental implants after increased awareness of tobacco use as a risk factor. *J Oral Maxillofac Surg* 1997; **55:** 72-75.

11. Esposito M, Hirsch J-M, Lekholm U, Thomsen P. Biological factors contributing to failures of osseointegrated oral implants. (I) Success criteria and epidemiology. *Eur J Oral Sci* 1998; **106:** 527-551.

12. Friberg B, Jemt T, Lekholm U. Early failures in 4,641 consecutively placed Brånemark dental Implants: a study from stage 1 surgery to the connection of completed prostheses. *Int J Oral Maxillofac Implants* 1991; **6:** 142-146.

13. Truhlar R S, Farish S E, Scheitler L E, Morris H F, Ochi S. Bone quality and implant design-related outcomes through stage II surgical uncovering of spectra-system root form implants. *J Oral Maxillofac Surg* 1997; **55:** 46-54.

14. Rangert B R, Sullivan R M, Jemt T M. Load factor control for implants in the posterior partially edentulous segment. *Int J Oral Maxillofac Implants* 1997; **12:** 360-370.

15. Clelland N L, Lee J K, Bimbenet O C, Gilat A. Use of an axisymmetric finite element method to compare maxillary bone variables for a loaded implant. *J Prosthodont* 1993; **2:** 183-189.

16. Blomqvist J E, Alberius P, Isaksson S, Linde A, Hansson B-G. Factors in implant integration failure after bone grafting. *Int J Oral Maxillofac Surg* 1996; **25:** 63-68.

17. Pontoriero R, Tonelli M P, Carnevale G, Mombelli A, Nyman S R, Lang NP. Experimentally induced peri-implant mucositis. *Clin Oral Implants Res* 1994; **5:** 254-259.

18. Mengel R, Stelzel M, Hasse C, Flores-de-Jacoby L. Osseointegrated implants in patients treated for generalized severe adult periodontitis. An interim report. *J Periodontol* 1996; **67:** 782-787.

19. Ellegaard B, Baelum V, Karring T. Implant therapy in periodontally compromised patients. *Clin Oral Implants Res* 1997; **8:** 180-188.

20. Liljenberg B, Gualini F, Berglundh T, Tonetti M, Lindhe J. Composition of plaque-associated lesions in the gingiva and the peri-implant mucosa in partially edentulous subjects. *J Clin Periodontol* 1997; **24:** 119-123.

21. Quirynen M, Listgarten M A. The distribution of bacterial morphotypes around natural teeth and titanium implants ad modum Branemark. *Clin Oral Implants Res* 1990; **4:** 8-12.

22. Mobelli A, Marxer M, Gaberthuel T, Grunder U, Lang NP. The microbiota of osseointegrated implants in patients with a history of periodontal disease. *J Clin Periodontol* 1995; **22:** 124-130.

23. Quirynen M, Peeters W, Naert I, Coucke W, Van Steenbergeh D. Peri-implant health around screw-shaped c.p. titanium machined implants in partially edentulous patients with or without ongoing periodontitis. *Clin Oral Implants Res* 2001; **12:** 589-594.

24. Krekeler G, Schilli W, Diemer J. Should the exit of the artificial abutment tooth be positioned in the region of the attached gingival? *Int J Oral Surg* 1985; **14:** 504-508.

25. Artizi Z, Tal H, Moses O, Kozlovsky A. Mucosal considerations for osseointegrated implants. *J Prosthet Dent* 1993; **70:** 427-432.

26. Warrer K, Buser D, Lang N P, Karring T. Plaque-induced peri-implantitis in the presence or absence of keratinised mucosa. *Clin Oral Implants Res* 1995; **6:** 131-138.

27. Esposito M, Hirsch J-M, Lekholm U, Thomsen P. Biological factors contributing to failures of osseointegrated oral implants (II). Etiopathogenesis. *Eur J Oral Sc* 1998; **106:** 721-764.

28. Marx R E, Johnson R P. Studies in the radiobiology of osteoradionecrosis and their clinical significance. *Oral Surg Oral Med Oral Pathol Oral Radiol Endod* 1987; **64:** 379-390.

29. Coulthard P, Esposito M, Worthington H V, Jokstad A. Interventions for replacing missing teeth: hyperbaric oxygen therapy for irradiated patients who require dental implants. (Cochrane Review) *In: The Cochrane Library 2002, Issue 3.* Oxford: Update Software

30. Eriksson A R, Albrektsson T. Temperature threshold levels for heat-induced bone tissue injury: A vital microscopic study in the rabbit. *J Prosthet Dent* 1983; **50:** 101-107.

31. Lyer S, Weiss C, Mehta A. Effects of drill speed on heat production and quality of bone formation in dental implant osteotomies. Part II: relationship between drill speed and healing. *Int J Prosthodont* 1997; **10:** 536-540.

32. Naert I, Quirynen M, Van Steenberghe D, Darius P. A study of 589 consecutive implants supporting complete fixed prostheses. Part II: Prosthetic aspects. *J Prosthet Dent* 1992; **68:** 949-956.

33. Esposito M, Coulthard P, Worthington H V, Jokstad A. Interventions for replacing missing teeth: different types of dental implants. (Cochrane Review) *In: The Cochrane Library 2002, Issue 4.* Oxford: Update Software

34. Smith R A, Berger R, Dodson T B. Risk factors associated with dental implants in healthy and medically compromised patients. *Int J Oral Maxillofac Implants* 1992; **7:** 367-372.

35. Van Steenberghe D, Lekholm U, Bolender C, Folmer T, Henry P, Herrmann I, Higuchi K, Laney W, Linden U, Åstrand P. The applicability of osseointegrated oral implants in the rehabilitation of partial edentulism: A prospective multicenter study on 558 fixtures. *Int J Oral Maxillofac Implants* 1990; **5:** 272-281.

36. Nishioka G J, Jones J, Triplett R G, Aufdemorte T B. The role of bacterial-laden biofilms in infections of maxillofacial biomaterials. *J Oral Maxillofac Surg* 1988; **46:** 19-25.

37. Costerton J W, Irvin R T, Cheng K-J. The bacterial glycocalyx in nature and disease. *Ann Rev Microbiol* 1981; **35:** 299-324.

38. Melcher G A, Hauke C, Metzdorf A, Perren G, Schilegel U, Ziegler W J. Infection after intramedullary nailing: An experimental investigation on rabbits. *Injury* 1996; **27:** SC23-26.

39. Deporter D A, Freidland B, Watson P A, Pilliar R M, Howley T P, Abdulla D, Melcher A H, Smith D C. A clinical and radiographic assessment of a porous-surfaced, titanium alloy dental implant system in dogs. *Int J Oral Implantol* 1987; **4:** 31-37.

40. Laskin D M, Dent C D, Morris H F, Ochi S, Olson J W. The influence of preoperative antibiotics on success of endosseous implants at 36 months. *Ann Periodontol* 2000; **5:** 166-174.

41. Lambert P M, Morris H F, Ochi S. The influence of 0.12% chlorhexidine digluconate rinses on the incidence of infectious complications and implant success. *J Oral Maxillofac Surg* 1997; **55:** 25-30.

42. Balshi T J, Wolfinger G J. Immediate loading of Brånemark implants in edentulous mandibles: a preliminary report. *Implant Dent* 1997; **6:** 83-88.

43. Schnitman P A, Wohrle P S, Rubenstein J E, Dasilva J D, Wang N-H. Ten-year results for Brånemark implants immediately loaded with fixed prostheses at implant placement. *Int J Oral Maxillofac Implants* 1997; **12:** 495-503.

44. Goodman S, Wang J-S, Doshi A, Aspenberg P. Difference in bone ingrowth after one versus two daily episodes of micromotion: experiments with titanium chambers in rabbits. *J Biomed Mater Res* 1993; **27:** 1419-1424.

45. Goodman S B. The effects of micromotion and particulate materials on tissue differentiation. Bone chamber studies in rabbits. *Acta Orthop Scand* 1994; **65:** 1-43.

46. Branemark P-I, Engstrand P, Ohrnell L-O, Grondahl K, Nilsson P, Hagberg K, Darle C, Leckholm U. Branemark Novum: a new treatment concept for the rehabilitation of the edentulous mandible. Preliminary results from a prospective clinical follow-up study. *Clin Implant Dent Rel Res* 1999; **1:** 2-16.

47. Roccuzzo M, Bunino M, Prioglio F, Bianchi S D. Early loading of sandblasted and acid-etched (SLA) implants: a prospective split-mouth comparative study. *Clin Oral Implants Res* 2001; **12:** 572-578.

48. Esposito M, Worthington H V, Coulthard P, Jokstad A. Interventions for replacing missing teeth: different times for loading dental implants (Cochrane Review) *In: The Cochrane Library* 2003, *Issue 1.* Oxford: Update Software

49. Cochran D. Implant therapy I. *Ann Periodont* 1996; **1:** 707-790.

50. Strub J R, Witkowski S, Einele F. Prosthodontic aspects of implantology. *In:* Watzek G (ed) *Endosseous implants: scientific and clinical aspects.* Chicago: Quintessence Books. p319-407.

51. Skalak R. Biomechanical considerations in osseointegrated prostheses. *J Prosthet Dent* 1983; **49:** 843-848.

52. Shackleton J L, Carr L, Slabbert J C G, Becker P J. Survival of fixed implant-supported prostheses related to cantilever lengths. *J Prosthet Dent* 1994; **71:** 23-26.

53. Tricia J, Laohapand P, Van Steenberghe D, Quirynen M, Naert

l. Mechanical state assessment of the implant bone continuum: A better understanding of the periotest method. *Int J Oral Maxillofac Implants* 1995; **10:** 43-49.

54. Sullivan D Y, Sherwood R L, Collins T A, Krogh P H J. The reverse-torque test: A clinical report. *Int J Oral Maxillofac Implants* 1996; **11:** 179-185.

55. Meredith N, Alleyne D, Cawley P. Quantitative determination of the stability of the implant-tissue interface using resonance frequency analysis. *Clin Oral Implants Res* 1996; **7:** 262-267.

56. Elias J J, Brunski J B, Scarton H A. A dynamic model testing technique for non-invasive assessment of bone-dental implant interfaces. *Int J Oral Maxillofac Implants* 1996; **11:** 728-734.

57. Frederiksen N L. Diagnostic imaging in dental implantology. *Oral Surg Oral Med Oral Pathol Oral Radiol Endod* 1995; **80:** 540-554.

58. Bragger U. Radiographic parameters for the evaluation of peri-implant tissues. *Periodontol* 2000; **4:** 87-97.

59. Grondahl M, Lekholm U. The predictive value of radiographic diagnosis of implant instability. *Int J Oral Maxillofac Implants* 1997; **12:** 59-64.

60. Albrektsson T, Zarb G, Worthington P, Eriksson A R. The long-term efficacy of currently used dental implants. A review and proposed criteria of success. *Int J Oral Maxillofac Implants* 1986; **1:** 11-25.

61. Quirynen M, Naert I, Van Steenberghe D, Dekeyser C, Callens A. Periodontal aspects of osseointegration fixtures supporting a partial bridge. An up to 6-year retrospective study. *J Clin Periodontol* 1992; **19:** 118-126.

62. Esposito M, Worthington H V, Coulthard P, Jokstad A. Interventions for replacing missing teeth: maintaining and re-establishing health around dental implants. (Cochrane Review). *In: The Cochrane Library* 2002, *Issue 3.* Oxford: Update Software.

63. Albrektsson T, Isidor F. Consensus report of session IV. In: Lang NP, Karring T Eds *Proceedings of the 1st European Workshop on Periodontology.* London: Quintessence Pubishing Co Ltd 1994;365-369.

64. Mombelli A. Prevention and therapy of peri-implant infections. *In:* Lamg N P, Karring T, Lindhe J (eds) *Proceedings of the 3rd European Workshop on Periodontology* pp 281-303. 1999 Berlin: Quintessence Books.

65. Rosenberg E S, Torosian J P, Slots J. Microbial differences in 2 clinically distinct types of failures of osseointegrated implants. *Clin Oral Implants Res* 1991; **2:** 135-144.

66. Augthun M, Conrads G. Microbial findings of deep peri-implant bone defects. *Int J Oral Maxillofac Implants* 1997; 12:106-112.

67. Esposito M, Hirsch J-M, Leckholm U, Thomsen P. Differential diagnosis and treatment strategies for biological complications and failing oral implants. A review of the literature. *Int J Oral Maxillofac Implants* 1999; **14:** 473-490.

68. Orton G O, Steele D L, Wolinsky L E. The dental professional's role in monitoring and maintenance of tissue-integrated prostheses. *Int J Oral Maxillofac Implants* 1989; **4:** 305-310.

69. Quirynen M, De Soete M, van Steenberghe D. Infectious risks for oral implants: a review of the literature. *Clin Oral Impl Res* 2002; **12:** 1-19.

70. Lang N P, Adler R, Joss A, Nyman S. Absence of bleeding on probing. An indicator of periodontal stability. *J Clin Periodontol* 1990; **17:** 714-721.

71. Lang N P, Mombelli A, Bragger U, Hammerle CH. Monitoring disease around dental implants during supportive periodontal treatment. *Periodontol* 2000; **12:** 60-68.

72. Schou S, Holmstrup P, Stoltze K, Hjorting-Hansen E, Fiehn N E, Skovgaard L T. Probing around implants and teeth with healthy or inflamed peri-implant mucosa/gingival. *Clin Oral Implants Res* 2002; **13:** 113-126.

73. Orton G O, Steele D L, Wolinsky L E. The professional's role in monitoring and maintenance of tissue-integrated prostheses. *Int J Oral Maxillofac Implants* 1989; **4:** 305-310.

74. Bragger U. Maintenance, monitoring, therapy of implant failures. *In:* Lang NP, Karring T (eds) Proceedings of the 1st European Workshop on Periodontology. London: Quintessence Publishing Co Ltd, 1994, 345-364.

75. Meffert R M. Chemotherapeutic mouthrinses as adjuncts in implant dentistry. *Am J Dent* 1989; **2:** 317-321.

76. Garber D A. Implants — the name of the game is still maintenance. *Compend Contin Educ Dent* 1991; **12:** 876-886.

77. Wolff L, Kim A, Nunn M, Bakdash B, Hinrichs J. Effectiveness of a sonic toothbrush in maintenance of dental implants. A prospective study. *J Clin Periodontol* 1998; **25:** 821-828.

78. Fox S C, Moriarty J D, Kusy R P. The effects of scaling a titanium implant surface with metal and plastic instruments: an *in vitro* study. *J Periodontol* 1990; **61:** 485-490.

79. Dmytryk J J, Fox S C, Moriarty J D. The effects of scaling titanium implant surfaces with metal and plastic instruments on cell attachment. *J Periodontol* 1990; **61:** 491-496.

80. Lavigne S E, Krust-Bray K S, Williams K B, Killoy W J, Theisen F. Effects of subgingival irrigation with chorhexidine on the periodontal status of patients with HA-coated Integral dental implants. *Int J Oral Maxillofac Implants* 1994; **9:** 156-162.

81. Strooker H, Rohn S, Van Winkelhoff A J. Clinical and microbiologic effects of chemical versus mechanical cleansing in professional supportive implant therapy. *Int J Oral Maxillofac Implants* 1998; **13:** 845-850.

82. Mombelli A, Lang N P. Antimicrobial treatment of peri-implant infections. *Clin Oral Implants Res* 1992; **3:** 162-168.

83. Mouhyi J, Sennerby L, Pireaux J-J, Dourov N, Nammour S, Van Reck J. An XPS and SEM evaluation of six chemical and physical techniques for cleaning of contaminated titanium implants. *Clin Oral Implants Res* 1998; **9:** 185-194.

84. Bach G, Neckel C, Mall C, Krekeler G. Conventional versus laser-assisted therapy of peri-implantitis: a five-year comparative study. *Implant Dent* 2000; **9:** 247-251.

85. Von Arx T, Kurt B, Hardt N. Treatment of severe peri-implant bone loss using autogenous bone and a resorbable membrane. Case report and literature review. *Clin Oral Implants Res* 1997; 8: 517-526.

86. Esposito M, Worthington H V, Coulthard P. In search of the truth: the role of systematic reviews and meta-analyses for assessing the effectiveness of rehabilitation with oral implants. *Clin Implant Dent Rel Res* 2001; **3:** 62-78.

87. Esposito M, Coulthard P, Worthington H V, Jokstad A. Quality assessment of randomised clinical trials of oral implants. *Int J Oral Maxillofac Implants* 2001; **16:** 783-792.

IN BRIEF

- Ageing dentate patients are increasing in number.
- Caries risk assessment facilitates dental management.
- Restoration monitoring, repair or refurbishment should always be considered before a restoration is placed.
- Stabilisation splints are helpful in preventing further non-carious tooth tissue loss.
- Fluoride release from restorative materials may not have a therapeutic benefit.
- Dry mouth is not specifically age related.

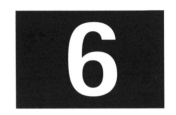

Prevention. Part 6: Prevention in the older dentate patient

P. A. Brunton[1]; Series Editor E. J. Kay[2]

Managing the ageing dentition is a frequent problem for practitioners. Prevention of further tooth loss, let alone preserving tooth tissue, whilst minimising the effects of operative intervention form the basis for successful management of older dentate patients. The purpose of this article is to consider the prevention of caries, further tooth tissue loss due to operative intervention and non-carious tooth tissue loss in the ageing dentate patient.

PREVENTION

[1]*Senior Lecturer/Honorary Consultant in Restorative Dentistry, Unit of Integrated Restorative Care, University Dental Hospital of Manchester, Higher Cambridge Street, Manchester M15 6FH;
[2]Professor of Dental Health Services Research, University of Manchester Dental Hospital and School, Higher Cambridge Street, Manchester M15 6FH
*Correspondence to: Dr Paul A. Brunton
E-mail: paul.brunton@man.ac.uk

Last scene of all,
That ends this strange eventful history,
Is second childishness and mere oblivion,
Sans teeth, sans eyes, sans taste, sans everything
  As You Like It, Shakespeare (c.1599)

Twenty years ago Shakespeare's vision of ageing in the UK was alarmingly accurate with people commonly surviving their natural dentition. Advances in our understanding of dental disease and dental care coupled with increasing dental awareness and motivation by patients has fortunately changed his somewhat dim view of dental ageing.

The part played by the dental profession in this public health success story is sadly somewhat underplayed. One of the consequences of our success however, which practitioners face on a day-to-day basis is managing the ageing dentition. This along with meeting the expectations of an ever increasing elderly population with quite rightly youthful expectations of both function and aesthetics is demanding. Prevention of further tooth tissue and tooth loss *per se* is paramount in the management of all patients but especially elderly dentate patients. One retained tooth, for example, can support and help retain a lower partial denture with which the patient can function whereas a complete lower denture would be unstable with poor retention, particularly if the ridge is especially atrophic.

Caries is often described as a disease of the two extremes of life assuming all risk factors remain equal. The availability of fluoride in toothpaste particularly has changed the pattern of disease seen by practitioners, with caries largely confined to pits and fissures and smooth surface caries relatively uncommon in younger patients. In contrast elderly patients are more likely to present with root caries and caries adjacent to existing restorations. Alongside this different pattern of caries experience elderly patients present with non-carious tooth tissue loss, the cumulative effects of generalized periodontitis and failing often quite advanced restorative dentistry.

The purpose of this article is to consider the prevention of caries, further tooth tissue loss due to operative intervention and non-carious tooth tissue loss in the elderly dentate patient. Prevention for the edentulous patient with or without implant-retained prostheses is covered elsewhere in the series. Many of the interventions we prescribe for our patients on a daily basis are not evidence-based and considerable research is required to provide an evidence base for our clinical practice. There are however a lack of clinical studies in this area, which makes this difficult. Given the increasing number of elderly dentate patients it is suggested that this is an area that deserves some priority when research funding is allocated. Interventions suggested for

Caries risk assessment

Helps the practitioner decide whether to intervene and informs the frequency of subsequent recall and radiographs

prevention in the elderly dentate patient will however be supported by evidence where it is available. The strength of this evidence will be indicated using the following hierarchy of evidence:

Type 1 Systematic review of at least one randomized controlled trial (RCT)
Type 2 At least one RCT
Type 3 Non-randomized intervention studies
Type 4 Observational studies
Type 5 Traditional reviews, expert opinion

CARIES
Caries is a totally preventable disease irrespective of a patient's age. Assuming all risk factors remain equal it is unusual to see new lesions in any patient but particularly in older patients where susceptible pits and fissures if prone to caries will already have experienced the disease. Physiological ageing of a dentition however results in gradual exposure of root surfaces, which can be prone to caries in later life ie a new susceptible site emerges and consequently the pattern of disease experience changes with age.

Currently there is considerable debate in the literature regarding the management of dental caries with the evidence suggesting that we move to a less interventive approach. This involves concentrating our efforts on arresting established lesions, especially root and cervical caries, reversing early occlusal lesions and only intervening when lesions are cavitated. Central to this philosophy is assessing the caries risk of our patients and recognizing that this assessment can change.

Patients can move from low to high risk by changing their diet, for example, older patients post radiotherapy or past smokers sucking sweets more frequently than normal to combat the effects of a dry mouth or in lieu of a cigarette.

Restricting operative intervention to high and moderate risk patients whilst opting for a preventive monitoring type approach in low risk patients is arguably a more scientific approach to the management of the dental caries rather than the purely surgical approach traditionally adopted in the UK.

ASSESSING CARIES RISK
Caries risk assessment is defined as the risk that a patient will develop new lesions of caries or existing lesions will continue to progress assuming that all aetiological factors (diet, time, susceptible surface and plaque levels) remain equal (Table 1). Individuals are assessed as being at high, medium and low risk of developing further lesions. A high-risk category would be allocated to a patient where the majority of the factors in Table 1 point to a high risk and vice versa. Moderate risk would be attributed where the factors in the table balance out.

It is an important assessment as it informs the recall period for patients in regular dental care, helps the practitioner to decide whether to intervene or instigate preventive regimes; let alone the frequency that further radiographs should be taken for monitoring purposes (Table 2). It is accepted however that the recommendations in Table 2 have no robust evidence base. A systematic review looking at the evidence base for 6-monthly check-ups is currently ongoing. Until such time as the results of this review have been reported it is suggested that the recommendations in Table 2 are a good starting point. Computer programs are available to help clinicians assess caries risk and also to plan preventive treatments but these systems are in their infancy and have yet to be fully evaluated.

CARIES PREVENTION
Having decided what the patient's caries risk assessment status is it is suggested that the following preventive regimes, which combine the application of fluoride and chlorhexidine (Type 2)[1] are appropriate:[2]

High Risk
High-risk patients require intensive prevention regimes to include:

- Baseline radiographs
- Prophylaxis with application of chlorhexidine for 1 minute followed by rinsing
- Apply sealant to pits and fissures, which must be checked for integrity at recall
- Fluoride varnish application. Patient should be advised not brush or eat hard foods for 10 hours. Three applications of fluoride varnish are recommended over a 3-month period
- Brushing twice a day with a fluoridated toothpaste

Table 1 Determination of caries risk

High	Factor	Low
Diet high in fermentable carbohydrate	**Diet** Check with diet history	Diet low in fermentable carbohydrates
Frequent consumption not confined to mealtimes	**Frequency** Check frequency of consumpton with diet history	Infrequent consumption or confined to mealtimes
High plaque score	**Plaque** Amount and nature	Low plaque score
Low flow rates High lactobacilli and streptococcus counts	**Saliva** Amount and nature	High flow rates Low lactobacilli and streptococcus counts
Not dentally motivated Deprived background Low dental aspirations High caries family	**Socio-economic Status**	Dentally motivated patients Privileged background High dental aspirations Low caries family
High number of Filled and Missing Surfaces (FMS)	**Past Disease Experience**	Low number of Filled and Missing Surfaces (FMS)
High number of Decayed surfaces (DS)	**Current Disease Experience**	Low number of Decayed surfaces (DS)
Irregular and/or pain only attenders	**Attendance Pattern**	Regular attenders
Infrequent use of rinses and toothpaste Non-fluoridated water supply	**Fluoride and Chlorhexidine**	Frequent use of rinses and toothpastes Fluoridated water supply
Xerostomia, Learning difficulties Cariogenic medication	**Medical History**	Fit and well
Partial dentures used to replace missing units	**Other**	Bridgework used to replace missing units

- Rinsing daily for 1 minute with a fluoride mouthwash (0.05% NaF) at bedtime (Type 2)[3]
- Rinse weekly rather than daily (Type 2)[4] with a chlorhexidine solution for 6 weeks
- After 6 months repeat baseline radiographs to monitor proximal lesions and restore any lesions, which have reached the middle third of dentine. If progression has been detected increase the application of chlorhexidine and apply fluoride varnish two to three times on a six monthly basis
- Oral hygiene instruction and dietary counseling are required to ensure success
- Monitor patient at six monthly intervals until patient's caries risk falls to moderate or low

Moderate risk
Prevention for patients in this group should include:

- Prophylaxis followed by fluoride varnish application. Patient should be advised not to brush or eat hard foods for 10 hours. Three applications of fluoride varnish are recommended over a 3-month period for every year the patient remains at moderate risk
- Brushing twice a day with a fluoridated toothpaste
- Rinsing daily for 1 minute with a fluoride mouthwash (0.05% NaF) at bedtime (Type 2)[3]
- Monitor lesion size and depth and whether new lesions arise at 6–12 monthly intervals until the caries risk moves to low. If lesions progress or new lesions arise increase applications of the fluoride varnish and give further dietary advice

Low risk
Prevention is limited to brushing twice a day with fluoridated toothpaste with reviews at 12–18 month intervals to check for white spot formation and proximal radiolucencies.

PRESERVING TOOTH TISSUE
Elderly patients if prone to caries in their youth are likely to have relatively large restorations, as a consequence of the restorative cycle or staircase, and these will be prone to eventual failure.[5] The term staircase is to be preferred as the word cycle implies a return to the start where clearly each step on the staircase is a step further to the loss of a tooth. Newer elderly cohorts will have progressively more sound teeth, as operative intervention will have been restricted to where indicated, with minimal preparations and where modern adhesive materials will have been used. These patients will require different management strategies and this will pose a challenge for practitioners in the future.

Currently on average 60% of restorations placed by practitioners are replacement restorations that are deemed to have failed in clinical service.[6] The commonest reason cited for replacing restorations is secondary caries. There is considerable debate in the literature as to what constitutes secondary caries, ie is it

Table 2 Caries risk assessment

Caries Risk	Recall Interval	Intervention	Radiograph Frequency
High	Six Monthly	Yes	Six Monthly
Moderate	Six Monthly- Annually	Yes	Annually
Low	1-2 years	Monitor and attempt to arrest and reverse the lesions	1-2 years

recurrent caries or residual caries or is it a new lesion. It has been suggested that secondary caries is in fact a new carious lesion adjacent to an existing restoration. As such it should be treated as a primary lesion and more often than not the adjacent restoration does not warrant complete replacement therapy (Type 4).[7] Marginal defects are often misdiagnosed as secondary caries and restorations replaced needlessly. Similarly restorations are frequently replaced that could have been repaired, refurbished or simply monitored.

Replacement of restorations where a more preservative approach could have been adopted pushes the tooth further down the restorative staircase which if followed to its ultimate conclusion will result in tooth loss. Practitioners are encouraged therefore to minimize the nature and effect of operative intervention wherever possible.

NON-CARIOUS TOOTH TISSUE LOSS
Elderly patients frequently exhibit the effects of non-carious tooth tissue loss (NCTTL). NCTTL is often multi-factorial and is a combination of erosion (intrinsic and or extrinsic), abrasion and attrition. Extrinsic erosion due to acid present in the diet will on the whole affect the labial surface of the anterior teeth and to a lesser extent the occlusal surfaces of the lower permanent molars. Intrinsic erosion due to acid regurgitation (gastric acid) will usually affect the palatal surfaces of the upper teeth and on occasion the occlusal surfaces of the lower permanent molars. The effects of NCTTL are cumulative and irreversible but in a similar manner to periodontal disease the process has periods of disease activity and quiescence. Consequently in a patient who presents with NCTTL it cannot be assumed that the disease process is still active and some form of assessment is required. This usually involves taking study casts and comparing them with casts taken 6 months later to determine if the process is still ongoing. Dietary analysis is important to identify factors that might be responsible for the NCTTL the patient has experienced. Liaison with a medical practitioner should intrinsic erosion be diagnosed will also be necessary. Once a diagnosis is made the prime objective is to stabilize the disease process and prevent further tooth tissue loss before addressing the patient's functional, aesthetic or occlusal needs. A significant number of patients are successfully managed on preventive regimes with relatively few patients needing extensive advanced restorative therapy.

Restoration replacement

Consider restoration repair, refurbishment or monitoring in regular patients

Missing teeth

Replacement of missing units with bridgework is associated with less caries and periodontal disease than the use of removable partial dentures to replace missing units

PREVENTION OF NON-CARIOUS TOOTH TISSUE LOSS

It is very important that a correct diagnosis is made if appropriate preventive measures are to be effective, recognising that NCTTL can be multi-factorial. It would be sensible to liaise with the patient's medical practitioner, particularly if you suspect intrinsic erosion is responsible for the NCTTL the patient has experienced. It is helpful to explain to your medical colleague, in the referral letter, the association between eating disorders, reflux etc and NCTTL. It is also important to emphasise that reflux can often be asymptomatic and NCTTL can be the first sign of an underlying problem. A dietary history will be required if you suspect an extrinsic erosive cause and counselling the patient with regard to their dietary habits may be necessary.

Patients often attend with NCTTL seeking an assurance that the condition will not deteriorate and are happy if further NCTTL can be prevented. Unfortunately many patients are treated with extensive treatments, for example, a full mouth rehabilitation in a slavish attempt to restore teeth to their pre disease shape and contour. Whilst this is appropriate for a small number of patients a more preservative preventive philosophy is indicated for the majority of patients. A hard acrylic splint, in the form of a stabilisation splint, is very helpful to prevent further tooth tissue loss due to attrition and this is frequently the only treatment required. Patient compliance with splint wear can however be problematical and as teeth scarcely meet in the day, night time wear is all that is required. It may also be used as a diagnostic aid, particularly if an increase in the occlusal vertical dimension is planned subsequently. If abnormal occlusal loading is identified as an aetiological factor this will also need to be corrected, by a specialist, but only after a period of splint wear.

A stabilization splint is designed to have the following features:

• Even contact of all teeth in centric relation (retruded contact position – RCP)
• Protrusive and excursive guidance
• No non-working interferences

To produce a stabilization splint for a patient on a semi-adjustable articulator the laboratory will need the following:

• Full arch impressions
• Facebow record
• Centric and protrusive occlusal records

The splint may need to be relined with cold cure acrylic resin to improve the retention of the appliance and occlusal adjustment will typically be required. Frequently this is the only treatment required to stabilize a patient's dentition and prevent further tooth tissue loss. The evidence base for using splints in this way however needs to be tested in a properly conducted randomised controlled clinical trial.

If you have a patient who has a history of recurrent vomiting, for example, as in hiatus hernia advise the patient not to brush their teeth after vomiting. This is because tooth brushing will further abrade the eroded tooth tissue. To prevent tooth tissue loss counsel your patient to rinse with either 0.05% NaF rinse or alkaline mineral water. These will neutralise the effects of the acid and prevent further erosion and decrease subsequent sensitivity.

FURTHER REMARKS

Removing all the caries: Is this always necessary?

A randomised controlled study (Type 2)[8] has demonstrated that if dentine affected by caries but uninfected is sealed in it does not progress and lesions will arrest and burnout. With newer adhesive materials the prospect of reliably sealing affected but uninfected dentine within the centre of a preparation is achievable clinically. This will reduce the incidence of carious exposure of the pulp and could be termed preventive endodontic therapy.

Fluoride release from restorative materials: Is this useful?

Manufacturers often make claims about fluoride release from restorative materials. Whilst water fluoridation and the topical effects of fluoride in toothpaste are beyond question the therapeutic effects of fluoride release from restorative materials are questionable. A systematic review of the literature (Type 1)[9] showed no evidence of a preventive effect when fluoride-releasing restorative materials are used. Practitioners should therefore not place undue reliance on manufacturers' claims regarding fluoride release.

Replacing missing teeth: denture or bridgework?

In an elderly population who are retaining more of their natural dentition the replacement of missing units is a common clinical situation faced by practitioners. A randomised controlled trial (Type 2)[10] has clearly demonstrated that the replacement of missing units with bridgework is associated with less caries and periodontal disease than the prescription of partial dentures. The use of bridgework in suitably selected cases for the replacement of missing units is arguably therefore a more preservative approach to fixed prosthodontics in the elderly.

Dry mouth: An age-related phenomenon?

It is a myth that salivary flow reduces due to ageing.[11] Dry mouth is however common for elderly patients who are on medication, which reduces salivary flow due to autonomic effects. This can change a patient's caries risk and new lesions may develop consequently. Similarly patients who have had surgery to their salivary glands and or radiotherapy will have reduced salivary flow. These patients are best managed with a saliva substitute to ease the feeling of dryness. There are several on the market but it is sensible to prescribe one that contains fluoride. At least one randomised controlled trial has shown that 10% chlorhexidine varnish is useful for controlling root caries in adults with a dry mouth (Type 2).[12]

1. Luoma H, Murtomata H, Nuuja T, Nyman A, Nummikoski P, Ainamo J, Luoma AR. A simultaneous reduction of caries and gingivitis in a group of schoolchildren receiving chlorhexidine-fluoride applications. *Caries Res* 1978; **12:** 290-298.
2. Anusavice K. Management of dental caries as a chronic infectious disease. *J Dent Educ* 1998; **62:** 791-802.
3. Fure S, Gahnberg L, Birkhed D. A comparison of four home-care fluoride programs on the caries incidence in the elderly. *Gerodontol* 1998; **15:** 51-59.
4. Persson R E, Truelove E L, LeResche L, Robinovitch M R. Therapeutic effect of daily or weekly chlorhexidine rinsing on oral health of a geriatric population. *Oral Surg Oral Med Oral Pathol* 1991; **72:** 184-191.
5. Elderton R J. Restorations without conventional cavity preparations. *Int Dent J* 1988; **38:** 112-118.
6. Burke F J T, Cheung S W, Mjör I A, Wilson N H F. Restoration longevity and analysis of reasons for the placement and replacement of restorations provided by vocational dental practitioners and their trainers in the United Kingdom. *Quintessence Int* 1999; **30:** 234-242.
7. Mjör I A. The location of clinically diagnosed secondary caries. *Quintessence Int* 1998; **29:** 313-317.
8. Mertz-Fairhurst E J, Curtis J W, Ergle J W, Rueggeberg F A, Adair S M. Ultraconservative and cariostatic sealed restorations: results at year 10. *J Am Dent Assoc* 1998; **129:** 55-66.
9. Randal R C, Wilson N H F. Glass-ionomer restoratives: a systematic review of a secondary caries treatment effect. *J Dent Res* 1999; **78:** 628-637.
10. Budtz-Jorgensen E, Isidor F. A 5-year longitudinal study of cantilevered fixed partial dentures compared with removable partial dentures in a geriatric population. *J Prosthet Dent* 1990; **64:** 42-47.
11. Heft M W, Baum B J. Unstimulated and stimulated salivary flow rate in different age groups. *J Dent Res* 1984; **63:** 1182-1185.
12. Banting D W, Papas A, Clark C, Proskin H M, Schultz M, Perry R. The effectiveness of 10% chlorhexidine varnish treatment on dental caries incidence in adults with dry mouth. *Gerodontol* 2000; **17:** 67-76.

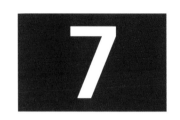

IN BRIEF

- Topical fluoride treatments are safe and effective but should be applied only to patients with decayed smooth surfaces or those at high risk of caries.
- Both APF gel and fluoride varnish are effective and can be recommended for caries prevention in permanent teeth. To maximize fluoride uptake, gels should be applied for 4 minutes.
- The frequency of fluoride application depends on individual risk, but should be at least biannual when indicated.
- Cleaning or prophylaxis is not necessary prior to the application of topical fluorides.

Prevention. Part 7: Professionally applied topical fluorides for caries prevention

R. Hawkins[1], D. Locker[2] and J. Noble[3]; Series Editor E. J. Kay[4]

This paper reviews the use of professionally applied topical fluorides (PATF) in caries prevention. PATFs are indicated for children and adults with one or more decayed smooth surfaces and/or those who are at high caries risk. Frequency of administration depends on the patient's caries risk, and is usually every 6 months. The effectiveness of fluoride varnish and gel applications has been well established in caries prevention trials involving permanent teeth. Although both types are effective, varnish may be preferred because it is easier to apply, reduces the risk of fluoride over-ingestion, and has greater patient acceptance. Fluoride foams are similar products to gels, but have not been tested clinically. The use of in-office two-part rinses is not recommended because they have not been proven effective. A cleaning, or prophylaxis, is not necessary before the application of topical fluoride for caries prevention. In conclusion, when used appropriately, PATFs are a safe, effective means of reducing caries risk among high-risk populations.

[1]Research Associate, [2]Director, [3]Research Assistant, Faculty of Dentistry, University of Toronto, Ontario, Canada; [4]Professor of Dental Health Services Research, University of Manchester Dental Hospital and School, Higher Cambridge Street, Manchester M15 6FH
*Correspondence to: Dr Robert Hawkins, Community Dental Health Services Research Unit, Faculty of Dentistry, University of Toronto, Room 521, 124 Edward Street, Toronto, Ontario, Canada M5G 1G6
E-mail: robert.hawkins@utoronto.ca

Caries prevalence among children in western countries has fallen dramatically over the past three decades.[1] Not all children, however, have experienced the same degree of caries risk reduction, and dental decay remains a significant problem for a substantial minority of high-risk children. The decline in caries prevalence has also not been uniform across tooth surfaces. On a percentage reduction basis, occlusal lesions have declined less than lesions on other tooth surfaces, and make up a higher proportion of the burden of dental caries.[2]

The use of professionally applied topical fluoride (PATF) is one means of preventing caries that is frequently used in private practice and public health settings. In terms of the relative reduction in decayed and filled surfaces, PATF is more effective against smooth surface caries than occlusal caries.[3] Given the present characteristics of dental caries, the appropriate use of PATF in developed countries must be examined.

Dental personnel have a wide choice of different PATF agents, vehicles, and regimens; and should be aware of the supporting evidence upon which to base their decisions. To gain a better understanding of the use of PATF, the following issues are reviewed: indications for use; caries prevention effectiveness and clinical application of different types of PATF; fluoride ingestion and toxicity; and whether a cleaning is necessary prior to topical fluoride application. The strength of the evidence was classified using the following typology:

Type 1: Systematic review of two or more clinical trials
Type 2: At least one randomized controlled trial
Type 3: Non-randomized intervention studies
Type 4: Observational studies
Type 5: Other designs, traditional literature reviews, expert opinion.

WHICH PATIENTS SHOULD RECEIVE PATF?

PATF should not be applied on a routine basis in dental practices. A patient's susceptibility to caries must first be determined and, based on this information an appropriate preventive care plan should be designed for each individual. The surfaces at risk for decay must also be considered because PATF is more effective against smooth surface caries than against pit and fissure caries.

Topical fluoride applications are indicated for patients with active smooth surface caries and those patients in high caries risk groups (Table 1). This includes special patient groups, such as those undergoing orthodontic treatment. In high-risk groups, evidence indicates an anti-caries effect over a 2-year period,[4] but PATF application does not make a significant difference in low-to-moderate risk children who also receive water fluoridation and dental sealants.[5,6] From a cost-effectiveness perspective, patients with low caries risk who reside in optimally fluoridated areas are unlikely to benefit from PATF therapy. The number of children that must be treated to prevent one decayed surface is esti-

Table 1 Indications for use of professionally applied topical fluorides

- Patients who are at high risk for caries on smooth tooth surfaces
- Patients who are at high risk for caries on root surfaces
- Special patient groups, such as:
  - Orthodontic patients
  - Patients undergoing head and neck irradiation
  - Patients with decreased salivary flow
- Children whose permanent molars should, but cannot, be sealed
- Not recommended for patients with low caries risk who reside in communities with optimal fluoridation

Biannual application of fluoride varnish can result in a reduction of 38% in caries increment over 2 years. Evidence available to date suggests that fluoride varnish and gel are equally effective in caries prevention

mated at 18 if caries incidence is low, but only 3 for groups with high caries incidence.[7]

A possible indication for the use of PATF is adults with exposed root surfaces. The problem of root caries is likely to increase due to population aging and the increased retention of teeth. However, no clinical studies have yet examined the potential benefits of this intervention.

FLUORIDE VARNISH

Since their introduction in the 1960s, fluoride varnishes have become the most widely used PATF in Europe.[8,9] The most common types of NaF varnish are Duraphat (2.2% F) and Fluor Protector (0.1% F). The advantage of varnish is its ability to adhere to tooth surfaces, which prolongs contact time between fluoride and enamel and improves fluoride uptake into the surface layers of enamel.

Caries prevention

For the permanent dentition, the anti-caries effect of fluoride varnish has been confirmed in a number of clinical trials. In a meta-analysis on the caries preventive effect of Duraphat varnish, eight studies were identified that were of high quality and provided Type 1 evidence.[10,11] Based on these studies, it was estimated the use of varnish resulted in a 38% reduction in caries increment (95% CI = 19–57%). In a second analysis, which included six additional studies, the estimated effect was again a 38% reduction (95% CI = 25–50%). Studies involved subjects ranging in age from 6-to-15 years; the application frequency was most often biannual; and the majority of studies were continued for at least 2 years.

Recent findings are consistent with the con-

clusions of the meta-analysis. In a high-risk community, children who received at least two varnish applications per year showed a 37% reduction in mean caries increment for a 4-year period compared with a control group.[12] Similarly, the effectiveness of fluoride varnish was supported in 24- and 48-month comparison studies of varnish and dental sealants.[13,14] In the 24-month report, compared with the control group, the use of fluoride varnish resulted in a 66% reduction in DMFS on non-fissured surfaces and a 38% reduction on fissured surfaces. However, in both reports, dental sealants were found to have superior performance for the prevention of decay.

The only direct comparison of the effectiveness of fluoride varnish and gel, in a developed country, showed no statistically significant differences between the treatment groups (NaF varnish and APF gel).[15] In this 3-year RCT study involving 12–13-year-olds, the mean total DMFS increments were 3.1 and 3.6 for the varnish and gel groups, respectively. The findings suggested varnish was as effective as gel for caries prevention.

For the primary dentition, the evidence is limited and only two randomized controlled trials have been conducted. Several studies of fluoride varnish have reported prevented fraction percentages of between 30-44%,[16,17] but findings have been inconsistent and most comparisons have not found significant differences. Recent studies have also found that varnish may slow the progression of early enamel caries in the primary dentition.[18,19] However, at present there is insufficient evidence with which to assess caries prevention effectiveness in primary teeth.

No definite conclusions can yet be drawn about the relative effectiveness of Duraphat and Fluor Protector varnishes.

Clinical application

PATFs must be reapplied at regular intervals to be effective and the frequency will depend on the risk level of the patient. Different application frequencies have been effective in clinical trials, but it is generally recommended that fluoride varnish be applied at least every 6 months.

The application of varnish is straightforward and can be done by a dental hygienist or a trained assistant (Table 2).[20] The entire process takes between 3–5 minutes per patient, depending upon the number of teeth present. Varnish is generally well accepted by dental personnel and patients, and has been found to be preferred to fluoride gel by both groups.[21] Dental hygienists found varnish easier and faster to apply, and allowed for better control of moisture and fluoride ingestion.

No common or serious side effects of varnish use have been reported. As a precaution, it is contraindicated in asthmatic patients due to possible allergic reactions. The temporary tooth discoloration caused by Duraphat varnish is objectionable to some patients, but is readily removed upon brushing.

Table 2 Procedure for the application of fluoride varnish

- Remove excess moisture from teeth with a cotton swab, cotton roll, or air syringe. Meticulous drying of the teeth is not necessary because the varnish will set in presence of moisture.
- Dispense 0.5–1 ml of varnish in a dappen dish. This should be enough for the entire dentition.
- Apply varnish as a thin layer using a disposable brush, or cotton pellet.
- The entire tooth surface must be treated, but do not place large amounts on tooth surfaces. Avoid applying varnish to gingival tissues because of the risk of contact allergies.
- No drying is required after application because varnish sets in a few seconds.
- The patient's mouth can be closed immediately following treatment.
- Patients can only have fluids or soft foods during the next four hours. Hard foods should be avoided.
- Patients should not brush their teeth for the rest of the day. This enhances the uptake of fluoride into the tooth structure.

Note: Varnish is contraindicated for persons with a history of allergies or asthma.

FLUORIDE GEL AND FOAM

Fluoride gel applications are more commonly used in the US and Canada. Gels are applied in Styrofoam mouth trays, and the most widely used gel is 1.23% F acidulated phosphate fluoride (APF). Fluoride foams are relatively recent products that are similar to gels, but have not been assessed in clinical trials.

Caries prevention

The effectiveness of PATF gels has been documented in numerous clinical studies. In a meta-analysis of fluoride gel trials, van Rijkom *et al.* included nine studies (ten comparisons) of professionally applied gels published between 1970 and 1992.[7] The overall average prevented fraction was 22% (95% CI = 18–25%) indicating good evidence of effectiveness in permanent teeth. All of the PATF studies used APF gel, application frequency varied from 1–2 times per year, and the ages of subjects ranged from 6–15 years.

No significant differences were found between application frequencies, but this result should be interpreted with caution because no head-to-head comparisons were included. Although two randomized trials have found no difference between annual and biannual application frequencies,[22,23] these studies could not control for the number of additional PATF applications which may have been received from private dentists not involved in the studies. Due to this possibility, there is a lack of evidence that annual applications are effective for caries prevention, and biannual applications are advisable.

A recently published Cochrane Review of fluoride gels included 25 studies, 14 involving PATF.[24] Based on these studies, the DMFS pooled prevented fraction was 28% (95% CI = 19–37%). The authors found insufficient information to evaluate application frequency, or caries prevention in the primary dentition.

Fluoride foams have not been assessed in clinical trials. Their characteristics are likely similar to gels because the same method of application is used, their fluoride concentrations are comparable, and fluoride enamel uptake is better.[25]

Clinical application

The frequency of gel application varies based on the caries risk level of the patient, and is usually provided at least every 6 months. Gel application is uncomplicated and can be performed by a dental auxiliary (Table 3).

The four-minute application of fluoride gel is recommended based on studies of enamel fluoride uptake.[26,27] When contact time is reduced to one minute, enamel fluoride uptake is significantly less. No clinical data support the 1 minute application of any product when used in the typical 6-month recall system. Nevertheless, many dental practices have reported applying fluoride gel for only 1 minute.[28]

Gel application is acceptable to most

Table 3 Procedure for the application of fluoride gel

- Mouth trays should be tried in the patient's mouth. It may be necessary to adapt or trim trays.
- Patient should be seated upright and suction should be used during the procedure.
- Teeth should be air-dried before gel application. For caries prevention, cleaning or prophylaxis is unnecessary prior to PATF.
- Enough gel, or foam, should be used to completely cover the teeth, but should be no more than 2–2.5 grams per tray or 40% of the tray's volume.
- Upper and lower trays should be inserted separately.
- Fluoride should be applied for 4 minutes, not 1 minute.
- Patient should expectorate for 1–2 minutes after tray removal.
- Patient should not rinse, eat, or drink for at least 30 minutes after the procedure.

Note: For patients with porcelain or resin restorations, neutral sodium fluoride is recommended to prevent etching of restorations.

patients. However, some children find the experience to be unpleasant, and gagging may occur with young children. The most common adverse effect is over-ingestion, which can lead to nausea and vomiting. The inadvertent ingestion of gel can be prevented by the use of a suction device, seating the patient upright, not overfilling trays, and using well-fitted trays.

IN-OFFICE FLUORIDE RINSES

Two-part fluoride rinses are being used more frequently in North American practices instead of gels or foams.[28] These rinses consist of two fluorides, APF and stannous fluoride, which are mixed or used concurrently; and are different from the mouthrinses used in school-based programs or home-use.[29]

Two-part rinses are marketed as a preventive agent that is better tolerated than tray applications and reduces fluoride ingestion. However, none of these claims has been supported. First, it is unlikely these products are as effective as other agents because the fluoride concentrations are much lower compared with APF gel (1,500–3,000 ppm vs. 12,300 ppm). Caries prevention effectiveness has not been reported in any randomized clinical trials. Second, the risk of ingestion is greater because rinses can be more easily swallowed. These rinses should never be used for young children because acute fluoride toxicity could result if they were swallowed. Lastly, it is doubtful whether in-office rinses are better tolerated by patients because of their sharp, metallic taste.

In-office fluoride rinses are not recommended for caries prevention because other effective anti-caries PATF products are readily available.

FLUORIDE INGESTION AND TOXICITY

Fluoride applications must be carefully monitored because the potential for overingestion and toxicity does exist. Fluoride is rapidly absorbed in the gastrointestinal tract and young children are particularly vulnerable. Patients should not be left unattended during the application of PATF.

A considerable amount of fluoride may be retained after gel application, even if suction

Studies of enamel fluoride uptake suggest that a four-minute application is to be recommended. Reducing contact time significantly reduces enamel fluoride uptake

PREVENTION

devices are used (on average 7.7 mg in children).[30] The risk of fluoride ingestion with fluoride foam is reduced, compared with gel, because a smaller amount is needed for applications. The exposure to and retention of fluoride foam by the patient may be significantly less compared with APF gel application.[25]

Fluoride varnish has a high fluoride concentration, but its safety is acceptable. Varnish is fast setting, fluoride is slowly released, and a small amount is needed for the complete dentition. Measurements of fluoride after topical treatments with varnish show levels far below those considered toxic.[31,32] Consequently, varnishes may be a better alternative to fluoride gels, especially for young children.[8]

PATF is not a risk factor for dental fluorosis when used at 6-month intervals, and if precautions are taken to minimize ingestion.[30]

IS A CLEANING NECESSARY PRIOR TO THE APPLICATION OF TOPICAL FLUORIDE?

Several clinical studies have reported that a cleaning, or prophylaxis, is not necessary before the application of topical fluorides.[23,33,34] No significant differences in caries reduction were found between patients who received a cleaning before application of PATF and those patients who did not receive a cleaning.

SUMMARY

The following is a summary of the important scientific facts and principles concerning the use of PATF:

- PATF should not be applied on a routine basis in dental practices. Fluoride applications are only indicated for patients with decayed smooth surfaces and those at high caries risk (Type 1)
- Both APF gel and fluoride varnish are effective and can be recommended for caries prevention in permanent teeth (Type 1)
- Frequency of PATF application will depend on

the risk level of the patient, but should be provided at least on a biannual basis when indicated (Type 1)
- For gel applications, gel should be retained in the mouth for 4 minutes (Type 5)
- During topical fluoride application, precautions must be taken to minimize fluoride ingestion (Type 5), and
- No cleaning or prophylaxis is necessary before the application of topical fluoride for caries prevention (Type 1)

Table 4 provides a comparison of the different types of PATFs considered in this review. Evidence indicates varnish and gel applications are similar in caries prevention effectiveness in permanent teeth. Although no clinical trials support the use of fluoride foam, it is likely to be equivalent to fluoride gel use for caries prevention. For several reasons, fluoride varnishes may be a better alternative to fluoride gels, particularly for young children. These reasons include reduced risk of fluoride over-ingestion, greater patient acceptability, and faster and easier application. The use of in-office two-part rinses is not recommended. When used appropriately, professionally applied topical fluorides are a safe, effective means of reducing caries risk among high-risk populations.

1. Anderson R J. Changes in dental caries experience of 12-year-old school children in two Somerset schools: a review after an interval of 30 years. Br Dent J 1995;**179**:125-129.
2. Li S H, Kingman A, Forthofer R, Swango P. Comparison of tooth surface-specific dental caries attack patterns in US schoolchildren from two national surveys. J Dent Res 1993; **72**:1398-1405.
3. Woodward G L, Lewis D W. The use of professionally applied topical fluorides in the North York Public Dental Program. Quality Assurance Report No. 8, Community Dental Health Services Research Unit, University of Toronto, 1995.
4. Olivier M, Brodeur J M, Simard P L. Efficacy of APF treatments without prior toothcleaning targeted to high-risk children. Community Dent Oral Epidemiol 1992; **20**: 38-42.
5. Bagramian R A. A 5-year school-based comprehensive preventive program in Michigan, U.S.A. Community Dent Oral Epidemiol 1982; **10**: 234-237.
6. Bohannan H M, Klein S P, Disney J A, Bell R M, Graves R C,

> A cleaning or prophylaxis is not necessary prior to the application of topical fluorides

Table 4 Comparison of professionally applied topical fluorides

	Caries prevention	Clinical application	Fluoride ingestion	Cost	Acceptability
Varnish	Effective in high risk children (permanent teeth)	Easy / Application time varies	Lowest risk / Moisture can be better controlled than gel or foam	Most expensive	Preferred by patients and hygienists, compared with gel
Gel	Effective in high risk children (permanent teeth)	Easy / Four-minute application time	% retained can be substantial / Procedure must be followed to reduce risk	Low cost	Well-tolerated by most patients, but varnish is preferred
Foam	Not clinically tested / Likely similar to gel	Easy / Four-minute application time	Risk of over-ingestion is less compared with gel	Low cost	Not formally assessed / Likely to be similar to gel
In-office two-part rinses	Not clinically tested	Most convenient	Greater risk of swallowing / Not recommended for young children	Least expensive	Not formally assessed

Foch C B. A summary of the results of the National Preventive Dentistry Demonstration Program. *J Can Dent Assoc* 1985; **51**: 435-441.

7. van Rijkom H M, Truin G J, van't Hof M A. A meta-analysis of clinical studies on the caries-inhibiting effect of fluoride gel treatment. *Caries Res* 1998; **32**: 83-92.

8. Bawden J W. Fluoride varnish: a useful new tool for public health dentistry. *J Public Health Dent* 1998; **58**: 266-269.

9. Beltran-Aguilar E D, Goldstein J W, Lockwood S A. Fluoride varnishes: a review of their clinical use, cariostatic mechanism, efficacy and safety. *J Am Dent Assoc* 2000; **131**: 589-596.

10. Helfenstein U, Steiner M. Fluoride varnishes: a meta-analysis. *Community Dent Oral Epidemiol* 1994; **22**: 1-5.

11. Helfenstein U, Steiner M. A note concerning the caries preventive effect of Duraphat. *Community Dent Oral Epidemiol* 1994; **22**: 6-7.

12. Zimmer S, Robke F J, Roulet J F. Caries prevention with fluoride varnish in a socially deprived community. *Community Dent Oral Epidemiol* 1999; **27**: 103-108.

13. Bravo M, Baca P, Llodra J C, Osorio E. A 24-month study comparing sealant and fluoride varnish in caries reduction on different permanent first molar surfaces. *J Public Health Dent* 1997; **57**: 184-186.

14. Bravo M, Garcia-Anllo I, Baca P, Llodra J C. A 48-month survival analysis comparing sealant (Delton) with fluoride varnish (Duraphat) in 6- to 8-year-old children. *Community Dent Oral Epidemiol* 1997; **25**: 247-250.

15. Seppa L, Leppanen T, Hausen H. Fluoride varnish versus acidulated phosphate fluoride gel: a 3-year clinical trial. *Caries Res* 1995; **29**: 327-330.

16. Holm A K. Effect of fluoride varnish (Duraphat) in preschool children. *Community Dent Oral Epidemiol* 1979; **7**: 241-245.

17. Twetman S, Petersson L G. Prediction of caries in pre-school children in relation to fluoride exposure. *Eur J Oral Sci* 1996; **104**: 523-528.

18. Peyron M, Matsson L, Birkhead D. Progression of approximal caries in primary molars and the effect of Duraphat treatment. *Scand J Dent Res* 1992; **100**: 314-318.

19. Autio-Gold J T, Courts F. Assessing the effect of fluoride varnish on early enamel carious lesions in the primary dentition. *J Am Dent Assoc* 2001; **132**: 1247-1253.

20. Blinkhorn A, Davies R. Using fluoride varnish in the practice. *Br Dent J* 1998; **185**: 280-281.

21. Warren D P, Henson H A, Chan J T. Dental hygienist and patient comparisons of fluoride varnishes to fluoride gels. *J Dent Hyg* 2000; **74**: 94-101.

22. Horowitz H S, Doyle J. The effect of dental caries on topically applied acidulated phosphate fluoride: results after three years. *J Am Dent Assoc* 1971; **82**: 359-365.

23. Johnston D W, Lewis D W. Three-year randomized trial of professionally applied topical fluoride gel comparing annual and biannual applications with/without prior prophylaxis. *Caries Res* 1995; **29**: 331-336.

24. Marinho V C C, Higgins J P T, Logan S, Sheiham A. Fluoride gels for preventing dental caries in children and adolescents (Cochrane Review). *In: The Cochrane Library, Issue 2, 2002.* Oxford: Update Software.

25. Whitford G M, Adair S M, McKnight C M, Perdue E C, Russell C M. Enamel uptake and patient exposure to fluoride: comparison of APF gel and foam. *Pediatr Dent* 1995; **7**: 199-203.

26. Wei S H Y, Hattab F N. Fluoride retention following topical application of a new APF foam. *Pediatr Dent* 1989; **11**: 121-124.

27. Wei S H Y, Lau E W S, Hattab F N. Time dependence of enamel fluoride acquisition from APF gels. II. *In vivo study. Pediatr Dent* 1988; **10**: 173-177.

28. Warren D P, Hensen H A, Chan J T. A survey of in-office use of fluorides in the Houston area. *J Dent Hyg* 1996; **70**: 166-171.

29. Ripa L W. Topical fluorides: a discussion of risks and benefits. *J Dent Res* 1987; **66**: 1079-1083.

30. Johnston D W. Current status of professionally applied topical fluorides. *Community Dent Oral Epidemiol* 1994; **22**: 159-163.

31. Ekstrand J, Koch G, Petersson L G. Plasma fluoride concentration and urinary fluoride excretion in children following application of the fluoride-containing varnish Duraphat. *Caries Res* 1980; **14**: 185-189.

32. Roberts J F, Longhurst P. A clinical estimation of the fluoride used during application of a fluoride varnish. *Br Dent J* 1987; **162**: 463-466.

33. Houpt M, Koenigsberg S, Shey Z. The effect of prior tooth cleaning on the efficacy of topical fluoride treatment: two-year results. *Clin Preven Dent* 1983; **5**: 8-10.

34. Ripa L W, Leske G S, Sposato A, Varma A. Effect of prior tooth cleaning on bi-annual professional acidulated phosphate fluoride topical fluoride gel-tray treatments: results after three years. *Caries Res* 1984; **18**: 457-464.

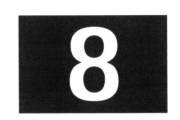

IN BRIEF

- Pit and fissure sealants are an effective preventive technology for children at high risk of dental decay as long as the sealant is retained.
- Autopolymerizing sealants and visible light curing sealants have high retention rates; glass ionomer cements have lower retention rates and their use is not recommended.
- Isolation of the tooth from contamination by saliva is the most important aspect of sealant placement.
- Cost-effectiveness requires that only those sites, surfaces and teeth at greatest risk should be sealed.

Prevention. Part 8: The use of pit and fissure sealants in preventing caries in the permanent dentition of children

D. Locker[1] and A. Jokovic[2]; Series Editor E. J. Kay[3]

This paper reviews evidence concerning the use of pit and fissure sealants in preventing caries in the permanent dentition of children. While the evidence with respect to some sealant types and application techniques is incomplete, systematic reviews have clearly demonstrated that sealants are an effective preventive technology when used in high risk children, and that with proper application techniques long-term retention rates can be achieved. However, careful selection of patients and teeth for sealant placement is required to ensure cost-effectiveness.

PREVENTION

1. Smoking cessation advice
2. Dietary advice
3. Prevention of tooth wear
4. Toothbrushing advice
5. Patients requiring osseointegrated oral implant treatment
6. Older dentate patient
7. Professionally applied topical fluorides for caries prevention
8. **Pit and fissure sealants in preventing caries in the permanent dentition of children**

[1]*Director, [2]Research Associate, Community Dental Health Services Research Unit, Faculty of Dentistry, University of Toronto, Ontario, Canada; [3]Professor of Dental Health Services Research, University of Manchester Dental Hospital and School, Higher Cambridge Street, Manchester M15 6FH
*Correspondence to: Dr David Locker, Faculty of Dentistry, University of Toronto, 124 Edward Street, Toronto, Ontario M5G 1G6, Canada
E-mail: david.locker@utoronto.ca

Over the past three decades there has been a substantial improvement in the oral health of children as evidenced by declines in the prevalence and severity of dental decay. Systematic exposure to fluorides, along with better nutrition, rising material standards of living and better access to dental care have reduced the susceptibility of contemporary child populations to infectious diseases affecting the oral cavity. For example, a recent study of Canadian children aged 13–14 years found that 64% were caries free.[1] However, among those with some experience of decay DMFT values ranged from 1 to 11 with a mean close to 3.0. This indicates that in this population a substantial minority remain susceptible to decay and that there is significant variation in the risk of disease among those who remain susceptible. For many of these children, effective caries preventive techniques are available which can reduce substantially their experience of this disease.

These preventive methods can be easily applied in dental practice and there is a substantial body of research evidence with respect to their effectiveness. For example, systematic reviews have been published for fluoride gel, fluoride varnish, chlorhexidine, pit-and-fissure sealants and dental health education.[2] This review summarizes the evidence for pit-and-fissure sealants when used to prevent caries in the permanent dentition of child populations. The rationale for the use of sealants as a major preventive intervention is the high prevalence of pit and fissure caries. Evidence suggests that between 90% of caries in children occurs in pits and fissures.[3]

The review considers the following questions:

- How effective are sealants in preventing dental caries in children?
- Which is the best sealant material to use?
- Does the placement technique have an influence on effectiveness?
- Which tooth and tooth surfaces should be sealed?
- How soon after tooth eruption should sealants be placed?
- Which children should receive sealants?

The strength of the evidence having a bearing on these questions can be classified using the following typology:

Type 1: Systematic review of two or more clinical trials
Type 2: At least one randomized controlled trial
Type 3: Non-randomized intervention studies
Type 4: Observational studies
Type 5: Other designs, traditional literature reviews, expert opinion

SEALANT MATERIALS

Since their inception, a number of types of sealants have been developed and tested for effectiveness. These differ according to the base material used, the method of polymerization and

PREVENTION

Table 1 Types of sealants evaluated in effectiveness studies

- Autopolymerizing
- Visible light curing
- Fluoride containing visible light curing
- Autopolymerizing glass ionomer cements
- Resin-modified (light-cured) glass ionomer cements
- Resin-bonded amalgam

Although rates of dental caries in children have declined, a substantial minority remain susceptible to the disease and there is significant variation in risk among those who remain susceptible. The majority of caries in children occurs in pits and fissures

whether or not they contain fluoride.[4] The types of sealants that have been assessed are summarized in Table 1.

EFFECTIVENESS OF SEALANTS

The effectiveness of sealants has been documented in numerous clinical studies. A systematic review published in the early 1990s found that the preventive fraction (PF), that is the proportion of occlusal decay prevented, among children receiving a one-time application of autopolymerizing sealant was 71%.[5] This preventive fraction PF is given by $(I_0 - I_1)/I_0$ where I_1 is the incidence of dental caries in the group treated with fissure sealants and I_0 is the incidence in the control group. Ultra-violet light polymerized sealant had a PF of 46%, but this 'first generation' product is no longer available. Although studies had been undertaken of visible-light cured sealants, none allowed the PF to be calculated so these were excluded from this review.

This original review was updated in 2001 by the inclusion of an additional five studies.[2] While only one of these used the split mouth design, they provide additional evidence of the effectiveness of autopolymerizing sealants and some evidence that visible-light cured resin sealants are also effective. A second review of studies also reported that there is good evidence that sealants are effective in high caries risk children as long as the sealant is retained.[3]

Since sealants are accepted as an effective preventive method, it is no longer ethically acceptable to compare the decay experience of teeth that are sealed with teeth that are not. Consequently, new sealant materials cannot be assessed in this way. Rather, since occlusal caries does not develop as long as the sealant remains adhered to the tooth, the length of time sealants are retained is now used as a surrogate measure of their effectiveness in preventing decay. Studies can be conducted on the relative caries preventive effect of two or more types of sealant since all teeth involved in the study are sealed. However, sealant longevity tends to be the most common outcome in this type of study.

WHICH IS THE BEST SEALANT MATERIAL TO USE?

Studies of the retention rates of different types of sealant are complicated by the fact that studies used different follow-up times. While autopolymerizing sealants have been observed for as long as 15 years, newer materials have only been subject to short-term follow-up. Since the highest rate of sealant loss occurs during the first year after application,[6] the calculation of annualized loss rates can mean that sealants observed for short periods of time can appear to be less effective. Nevertheless, currently available evidence indicates the following:[7]

- Autopolymerizing sealants have high long-term retention rates, with 60% of surfaces remaining covered after 5 to 7 years.

- Visible light curing sealants have retention rates similar to autopolymerizing sealants.
- Fluoride-containing visible light cured sealants have only been evaluated in short-term studies but have retention rates similar to autopolymerizing and conventional light cured sealants for the equivalent follow-up periods. Whether or not the incorporation of fluoride leads to further reductions in caries incidence or enhances the inhibition of incipient or inadvertently sealed hidden caries has not been determined.
- Retention rates for glass ionomer cements, both conventional and resin-reinforced, are significantly lower than that of resin based sealants and their use is not recommended.
- Since the probability of sealant failure is highest soon after placement for all types of sealant, they should be evaluated clinically for partial or total loss within 1 year of placement.

DOES THE PLACEMENT TECHNIQUE HAVE AN INFLUENCE ON EFFECTIVENESS?

A detailed description of current thinking regarding sealant application techniques is to be found in Waggoner and Siegal.[8] They describe the following steps:

Cleaning the pit and fissure surfaces

Before acid etching and sealant placement the tooth surface must be cleaned of plaque and other debris. Surfaces can be cleaned using a prophy cup or brush with or without pumice, with an explorer and forceful rinsing with water, with a toothbrush and toothpaste or by means of air abrasion. Where different cleaning methods have been compared, no differences in retention rates have been found. Although widening of fissures with rotary instruments has been recommended, current evidence does not conclusively support this practice. One disadvantage is that in most jurisdictions this means that hygienists and dental assistants cannot be given the task of sealant placement.

Isolation of the tooth

Complete isolation of the tooth from contamination by saliva is the most important aspect of sealant placement. Isolation by rubber dam or cotton rolls are equally effective and result in similar retention rates. Since teeth that are not completely erupted are difficult to isolate, sealants should not in most circumstances be placed on teeth until the occlusal surface is completely free of gingival tissue.

Etching the enamel surface

In order for the sealant to adhere the enamel surface needs to be etched, usually with an orthophosphoric acid liquid gel. Liquid and gel are equally effective in terms of surface penetration and sealant retention. Clinical studies indicate that a 15 second etch is adequate for sealant retention and no additional benefit received from longer etching times of 45 or 60 seconds. Studies comparing acid etching with air abrasion as a method of enamel preparation are inconclusive. While bond strengths are comparable, one study found higher rates of micro-leakage for air-abraded enamel. However, a recent study[9] found no difference in retention rates on enamel surfaces prepared by the two methods.

Rinsing and drying the tooth

Rinsing and drying times are not important as long as they are sufficient to ensure the complete removal of all etching material from the tooth surface.

Applying the sealant

All pits and fissures should be sealed. The placing of a bonding agent on the surface prior to the sealant does not appear to enhance retention rates.

Polymerization

In order to reduce contamination, it is generally recommended that the polymerization of light cured sealants is undertaken immediately after placement. However, one study suggested that allowing the sealant to sit on the tooth surface for 20 seconds prior to polymerization increased sealant penetration.[10] Clinical studies of the effect of this on retention rates have not been conducted.

Evaluation of the sealant

The sealant should be inspected to ensure complete coverage of the occlusal surface and the occlusion checked for interferences. Filled sealants tend to be thicker than unfilled sealants and are more likely to require adjustment after placement.

WHICH TEETH AND TOOTH SURFACES SHOULD BE SEALED?

There have been changes in the distribution and severity of dental caries in the permanent teeth of children. The prevalence has declined, progression of carious lesions has slowed so that cavitation occurs later in the course of the disease and teeth appear to remain at risk beyond the first few years after eruption. According to Rozier[11] dental caries is now a disease that affects selected sites of selected surfaces of selected teeth. Since sealant placement is relatively expensive, this means that only those sites/surfaces/teeth at greatest risk should be sealed.

The teeth and tooth surfaces at greatest risk for caries are the pits and fissures of molars. While it was initially considered that the first molars are at greatest risk of attack, epidemiological studies indicate that first and second molars are at equal risk and have a higher probability of decay than any other tooth type. Consequently, both first and second molars are the main candidates for sealants. Premolars are much less susceptible to decay than molars and are less likely to be candidates for sealants.

There is some evidence, although incomplete, that while the greatest risk for decay in molars appears to be 2 to 4 years after eruption, the pits and fissures of first permanent molars remain susceptible to primary decay into adolescence and beyond.[12] This evidence challenges early guidelines suggesting that teeth remaining caries-free for 4 or more years after eruption do not need to be sealed. Consequently, the length of time since eruption should not be the main factor determining the placement of the sealant. Rather, the patient's overall caries risk should be the main criterion employed.

Other tooth-level factors which should be taken into account in decisions to use sealants are:

Tooth morphology

Pit and fissure morphology has a significant influence on the risk of caries. Teeth with deep pits and fissures that catch an explorer are the best candidates for sealants while teeth with wide and easily cleaned grooves do not require sealing.

Status of the proximal surfaces of the tooth to be sealed

If a proximal restoration involves the pit and fissure surfaces it should not be sealed. If proximal caries is present a non-carious occlusal surface may be a candidate for a sealant if conservative procedures for managing the interproximal decay are feasible.

Caries status of the occlusal surface

Occlusal surfaces whose caries status is uncertain or surfaces where the caries is confined to the enamel can be sealed, since early lesions will not progress but will arrest as long as the sealant remains intact. Such tooth surfaces should be assessed at regular intervals to ensure the complete retention of the sealant. Where caries has progressed to dentine the tooth should be restored. Preventive restorations involving sealant materials or composites may be indicated.[13]

Eruption status

Since adequate isolation is needed for sealant retention to be ensured, it is generally recommended that sealants not be placed until the tooth is sufficiently erupted for the risk of contamination by saliva during sealant placement to be eliminated.

Overall caries activity

If the individual's caries history indicates that they are susceptible to pit and fissure caries, any caries-free pit and fissures of the teeth at greatest risk should be sealed. Susceptibility is usually indicated by the occurrence of one or more caries lesions per year.

WHICH CHILDREN SHOULD RECEIVE SEALANTS?

Since an increasing proportion of children are caries free significant effort has been devoted to

The caries preventive potential of sealants has been demonstrated in numerous studies. Sealant retention rates are now used as surrogate measure of their effectiveness in preventing decay

Retention rates for glass ionomer cements are substantially lower than that for resin based sealants and their use is not recommended. First and second permanent molars are at equal risk of decay and more likely to decay than any other tooth type. These are the main candidates for sealant application

Cost–effectiveness requires that only those children at high risk for caries should be considered for sealant application

developing methods for identifying those individuals at highest risk of caries. Cost-effectiveness requires that only those children at high risk should be considered for sealant applications. Numerous factors have been included in caries risk prediction models. However, none are totally accurate and given the variations in caries levels, and variations in risk factors between age cohorts, socio-economic and cultural groups and the fact that risk profiles are constantly changing, it is unlikely that a universally applicable model will be developed.[14] However, the majority of models include, as significant risk predictors:

- Caries history in the primary and permanent dentition, and
- Current level of caries activity

Consequently, these should be the main factors considered when assessing whether or not a child is likely to benefit sufficiently from sealants for their use to be considered cost-effective.

SUMMARY

Although the evidence having a bearing on all aspects of sealant use is incomplete and the strength of the evidence underlying some recommendations somewhat uncertain, a recent US Workshop on Guidelines for Sealant Use[15] and a Canadian evidence based care report[7] summarized some important scientific facts and principles:

- Sealants have been shown to be safe and effective in preventing dental decay in susceptible teeth and individuals (Type 1);
- In addition to preventing caries, sealants can arrest incipient decay (Type 2);
- Cost-effective use indicates that sealants should be placed on the pits and fissures of teeth at greatest risk (predominantly first and second permanent molars) in individuals susceptible to decay (Type 4);
- Children with previous or current caries experience should be considered for sealants (Type 3); others should not.
- Pit and fissure caries begins in childhood and can continue into adolescence and adulthood (Type 4).
- Sealants should be placed as early as possible after the occlusal surface is free of gingival tissue and up to 4 years after eruption (Type 3). Placement may be indicated beyond 4 years post-eruption depending upon the caries sus-

ceptibility of the individual (Type 4).
- Resin sealants should be used: autopolymerizing (Type 1) and light-cured (Type 2/3) have satisfactory retention rates. Glass ionomer cements should not be used (Type 2/3).
- Sealant use is technique sensitive; particularly with respect to moisture control (Type 3).
- Sealants should be evaluated clinically, especially when placed over incipient decay (Type 2).

The main principle underlying the use of sealants is that prevention is better than treatment. Sound, non-diseased teeth even though sealed are more valuable than properly restored teeth. Nevertheless, the indiscriminate use of sealants is not recommended. Maximizing the cost-effectiveness of this preventive technology is an important consideration.

1. Locker D. *Evaluation of Ontario's targeted dental screening program for schoolchildren.* Program Evaluation Report No. 7. Community Dental Health Services Research Unit, University of Toronto, 2002.
2. Rozier G. Effectiveness of methods used by dental professionals for the primary prevention of dental caries. *J Dent Educ* 2001; **65:** 1063-1072.
3. Weintraub J. Pit and fissure sealants in high-caries-risk individuals. *J Dent Educ* 2001; **65:** 1084-1090.
4. Duke S. Pit and fissure sealant materials. *Compendium* 2001; **22:** 594-596.
5. Llodra J, Bravo M, Delgado-Rodriguez M, Baca P, Galvez R. Factors influencing the effectiveness of sealants - a meta-analysis. *Community Dent Oral Epidemiol* 996; **21:** 261-268.
6. Ripa L W. Sealants revisited: An update of the effectiveness of pit and fissure sealants. *Caries Res* 1993; **27** (Suppl): 77-82.
7. Jokovic A, Locker D. *Evidence-based recommendations for the use of pit and fissure sealants in Ontario's public dental health programs.* Quality Assurance Report No. 21, Community Dental Health Services Research Unit, University of Toronto, 2001.
8. Waggoner D, Siegal M. Pit and fissure sealant application: updating the technique. *J Am Dent Assoc* 1996; **127:** 351-361.
9. Kanellis M, Warren J, Levy S. Comparison of air abrasion versus acid etch sealant techniques: six month retention. *Paediatric Dent* 1997; **7:** 81-86.
10. Chosak A, Eidelman E. Effect of time from application until exposure to light on the tag lengths of a visible light polymerized sealant. *Dent Materials* 1988; **4:** 302-206.
11. Rozier G. The impact of recent changes in the epidemiology of dental caries on guidelines for the use of dental sealant: epidemiological perspectives. *J Public Health Dent* 1995; **55:** 292-301.
12. Richardson P S, McIntyre I G. Susceptibility of tooth surfaces to caries attack in young adults. *Community Dent Health* 1996; **13:** 163-168.
13. Hassall D, Mellor A. The sealant restoration: indications, success and clinical technique. *Br Dent J* 2001; **191:** 358-362.
14. Hausen H. Caries prediction — state of the art. *Community Dent Oral Epidemiol* 1997; **25:** 87-96.
15. Siegal M, Kumar J. Workshop on guidelines for sealant use: preface. *J Public Health Dent* 1995; **55:** 261-262.

The scientific basis of oral health education

The scientific basis of oral health education

R S Levine OBE
General Dental Practitioner and Independent Scientific Adviser,
370 Alwoodley Lane, Leeds LS17 7DN

C R Stillman-Lowe
Independent Oral Health Promotion Adviser,
7 Broadwater Road, Twyford, Reading RG10 0EX

2004
Published by the British Dental Association
64 Wimpole Street, London, W1G 8YS

Acknowledgements

With the closure of the Health Education Authority in 2000, the future of *The Scientific Basis of Dental Health Education* was thrown into doubt. We are grateful to the Health Development Agency and the Dental Practice Board for commissioning and publishing a revised fourth edition of the document in 2001. The support of many professionals for a fifth edition, more widely available, was substantial, and to those who put the case forcefully to us, including the then Chair of the National Oral Health Promotion Group and the President of the British Dental Hygienists' Association, we are also indebted.

As with the previous editions, a considerable debt of gratitude is owed to the panel of expert advisers, including a number of new members as well as several who were involved in the earlier editions. They have been generous with their time and advice to help ensure that the document remains a consensus of expert opinion. For the first time, with this edition, a formal consultation process with a wide range of professional bodies and agencies has taken place to help shape and develop the book. We are grateful to all those who took the time and contributed to this, so that the book could reflect the needs of the whole dental team.

Preface

The first edition of *The Scientific Basis of Dental Health Education* appeared in 1976 and was a slim booklet with a green cover. It arose from a joint attempt by the British Association for the Study of Community Dentistry and the Health Education Council, who published it, to refine and standardise the advice given to the public and to ensure that such advice was scientifically sound. The need for this document grew from the problem of confusing and sometimes conflicting dental health education messages being provided by professional and commercial bodies. The strength of the original document was that it came from an independent and authoritative source and was based on a consensus of scientific opinion from a group of the leading dental experts of the day.

Over the intervening quarter century, the document grew through four editions to become one of the most widely used and accepted sources of information on dental health, both in the UK and abroad. Now, the emergence of a more formalised system of evidence-based clinical practice, together with an increased emphasis on evidence-based oral health promotion, has made it essential to completely recast it for the twenty-first century. This book introduces a simple system for indicating the level of scientific evidence supporting a series of key statements on oral health. Following consultation with government and a range of professional bodies, both the format and the style have been changed to increase its readability and value to a wider range of user groups. New topics have been included in response to requests and the changing pattern of oral health. There is also a new series of appendices. These include information on smoking cessation, general healthy eating and sensible drinking guidelines, the eruption dates of teeth, first aid for traumatised teeth and evidence-based dentistry websites, for those who wish to keep up-to-date with new developments. In keeping with the wider range of oral topics now included, the title of this new edition has been changed to *The Scientific Basis of Oral Health Education.* To keep the book within a reasonable length, however, it does not attempt to cover the full scope of oral health promotion: this is covered well by other textbooks, listed in the further reading section.

As before, it is hoped that this new edition will be used by dental schools dental postgraduate deans and directors to help standardise undergraduate and postgraduate teaching and by professionals complementary to dentistry, whose role within the dental team has developed significantly since 1976. Those involved in general healthcare, such as medical practitioners, school nurses, health visitors, midwives, dieticians and pharmacists also have a vital role to play in oral health promotion, and it is hoped that this publication will be of value to them. Oral health promotion staff in the community dental service frequently provide training for people who can influence health in the wider community, such as teachers, childcarers and peer educators, and they can safely rely on the messages in this book as the basis for their programmes. Finally, it must be recognised that oral health education material is provided by a wide range of agencies, including government and professional bodies, charities, and commercial organisations in the form of both patient education material and for product promotion, much of which is of the highest standard. This too should conform to agreed expert opinion and it is hoped that this publication will be of assistance to these bodies.

Above all, this document is offered in the sincere belief that oral health education is one of our most important responsibilities and must be approached with the same dedication and professional quality standards that are applied to the operative treatment of disease. Only by offering the public consistent and soundly based advice can we hope that health education messages achieve their intended function of enabling individuals to control and improve their own health, as part of a comprehensive programme of national and local public health initiatives designed to tackle the determinants of poor health.

Ronnie Levine and Catherine Stillman-Lowe

May 2004

A guide to using this book

The aim of this book is to provide a sound basis for giving information and advice on the main aspects of oral health. The summary that follows gives a brief overview of the main oral diseases and some other oral conditions, together with four key messages. These key messages are a consensus of expert opinion and should form the basis of all oral health advice given to the public.

Chapters 1 to 11 cover the various diseases that can affect the teeth and mouth as a whole together with information on their causes and means of prevention, including advice for the under 5s and older people.

Throughout this document, important statements are given at the end of each chapter in the form of key points. In order to indicate the level of supporting scientific evidence for each of these key points a simple scheme called Evidence Base is used:

- Evidence Base A: Statements supported by very strong evidence from pooled research data (meta-analysis) or systematic literature reviews.

- Evidence Base B: Statements supported by the majority of relevant research studies.

- Evidence Base C: Statements that cannot be supported by a substantial body of research evidence, but where there is a consensus of scientific and professional opinion to support the statement.

More detailed information on Evidence Base is given in Chapter 12, together with sections on health education and the nature of scientific evidence.

Contents

Summary

The two most common oral diseases are tooth decay, or dental caries and gum disease, properly known as periodontal disease. The principal cause of dental caries is the frequent consumption of sugars, mainly in confectionery, snack foods and soft drinks, acting on the layer of bacteria on the tooth surface, which we call plaque. The sugars are rapidly converted into acid by plaque bacteria and the build up of acid attacks the tooth surface causing a cavity and if untreated, destruction of the tooth with pain and possibly infection.

The common form of periodontal disease is caused by poor oral hygiene allowing bacteria in the form of plaque to build up round the necks of the teeth. The toxins released from plaque cause inflammation of the gums, a condition known as gingivitis. The later stage of periodontitis develops when the supporting bone around the teeth becomes progressively destroyed, so that the teeth become loose and painful. Smoking is now recognised as a related cause. Unlike tooth decay, which is usually a rapid process, periodontal disease can take many years to reach the stage where teeth become loose and may be lost. In the UK the annual cost to the National Health Service for the treatment of these two conditions now exceeds £2 billion.

Dental erosion appears to be an increasing problem, which causes wearing away of the surface of the teeth. The cause is usually acid in the soft drinks and juices increasingly being consumed by children and young adults, 50% of whom are now affected to some degree. Erosion can also be caused by gastric regurgitation, as can occur in pregnancy, or due to conditions such as hiatus hernia or bulimia.

There are many other diseases that occur in the mouth and there are some conditions arising elsewhere in the body that can have a visible effect within the mouth, such as pregnancy, anaemia and HIV infection (AIDS). The most life threatening oral disease is oral cancer. This condition is nearly as common as cervical cancer in the UK, with about 4,500 new cases each year, most being smoking or alcohol related. About half of these cases prove fatal, but early diagnosis greatly improves the chance of survival. Dental patients who wish to give up smoking should be offered appropriate support to do so.

Dental disease is not an inevitable part of life and research has shown that much can be prevented by changes in behaviour. Such changes require the knowledge and skills to make healthy choices and these in turn are influenced by social and economic pressures, both on individuals and communities. These factors may account for the persistence of high levels of dental caries in economically depressed communities.

Key messages

To promote good oral health there are four key messages:

1. Diet: reduce the consumption and especially the frequency of intake of drinks, confectionery and foods with sugars.

The consumption of sugars, both the frequency and the amount, is important in determining the rate of tooth decay. When sugars are consumed, they should be part of a meal rather than between meals. Snacks and drinks should be free of added sugars, whenever possible. The frequent consumption of acidic drinks (such as fruit juice, squashes or carbonated drinks) should be avoided to help prevent dental erosion.

2. Toothbrushing: clean the teeth thoroughly twice every day with a fluoride toothpaste.

Effective daily toothbrushing with a fluoride toothpaste is the best way of preventing both caries and periodontal disease. Other oral hygiene aids such as floss and interdental brushes are best used after they have been demonstrated by a dentist, therapist or hygienist. Thorough brushing of all tooth surfaces and gum margins twice every day is of more value than more frequent cursory brushing, and a gentle scrub technique should be advised. A small soft to medium texture toothbrush should be used to allow all tooth surfaces and gum margins to be cleaned easily and comfortably. Effective toothbrushing with a fluoride toothpaste will help control caries provided that the diet is also favourable.

3. Fluoride: fluoridation of the water supply is a safe and highly effective public health measure.

Water fluoridation should be targeted at communities with higher caries levels. Where it is not technically feasible other fluoride strategies should be employed, such as programmes to promote the use of fluoride toothpaste.

4. Dental attendance: have an oral examination every year.

Everyone, irrespective of age and dental condition, should have an oral examination approximately once a year so that cases of oral cancer or other oral diseases can be detected early and treated. This advice also applies to those without any natural teeth. Children and those at risk from oral disease, including smokers, may need to be seen more frequently, as advised by the dentist.

IN BRIEF

- Caries is caused by the action of sugars on the bacterial plaque covering the teeth. Evidence Base A
- Caries occurs when demineralisation of the tooth surface exceeds remineralisation. Evidence Base A
- The risk of developing caries can be reduced by avoiding sugars between meals and at bedtime. Evidence Base B
- The risk of developing caries can be reduced by brushing with a fluoride toothpaste twice daily. Evidence Base A
- Never leave infants with sugars-sweetened drinks in feeding bottles or cups, especially at bedtime. Evidence Base B
- Caries occurs in all populations and age groups but is more common amongst children and disadvantaged groups. Evidence Base A

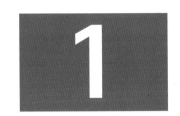

The scientific basis of oral health education. Part 1: Dental caries

R. S. Levine and C. R. Stillman-Lowe

WHO GETS CARIES?

This condition is often said to be the most common affecting mankind. This was true for much of the Western developed world during the previous century, but not for Asia and Africa. Within Europe and North America, the level of caries appeared to reach a peak in the 1960s and has decreased in prevalence during the past 30 years. Nevertheless it remains a major health problem for people of all ages. Its peak activity occurs during childhood. In the UK, national surveys are undertaken at regular intervals by the British Association for the Study of Community Dentistry. The 2001/2 national survey found at least one decayed tooth in 39% of 5-year-olds in England, 53% in Wales, and 55% in Scotland. The mean number of decayed teeth per child being, 1.47, 2.26 and 2.55 respectively.[1] In Northern Ireland in 1997/8, over 60% of 5-year-olds had caries experience, and the average number of decayed teeth per child was 2.9.[2]

There are wide variations in caries prevalence, often within small geographical areas and this is related to two social factors. Firstly, like many other diseases, it has become apparent that dental caries is essentially a disease associated with social deprivation. In the UK, low levels of caries can now be seen in the more affluent areas, especially in southern England. However, levels remain high in children in many inner city socially deprived areas of Wales, Scotland and Northern Ireland, and northern parts of England. The second factor is ethnicity and is a complex one, possibly related to different dietary and toothbrushing practices within different cultures. Some children of Asian ethnic background, including children of non-English speaking mothers, have the highest caries rates for deciduous teeth. One study of 5-year olds found that

Asian children had 60% more decayed teeth than white children living in the same towns.[3] However, this difference is not apparent in the permanent teeth of older children.

HOW CARIES AFFECTS TEETH

Dental caries affects the tooth itself. The consequences of caries are familiar to most people (Fig. 1)

The process begins at the tooth surface but is often hidden from sight in the fissures (grooves) or between the teeth. Where it is visible the initial appearance may be as a chalky white patch or ring around the neck of the tooth or as a shadow or staining on the biting surface (Fig. 2).

The chalky appearance is caused by the enamel surface having lost some of the calcium and phosphate mineral crystals of which it is largely composed. This process is called demineralisation. The destructive process can then spread into the dentine (the softer, sensitive part of the tooth beneath the enamel). The weakened enamel then collapses to form a cavity and the tooth is progressively destroyed. Caries causes progressive destruction of the crowns of the teeth often accompanied by severe pain and infection. The roots of teeth can also be attacked should they become exposed by gum recession and this is more common in older adults.

CAUSE

The basic process that causes caries is sometimes called an 'acid attack'.

Caries begins within the plaque on the tooth surface following the consumption of sugars in drinks and foods.

When sugars enter the mouth they are rapidly absorbed by the bacteria in the plaque layer on the surfaces of the teeth.

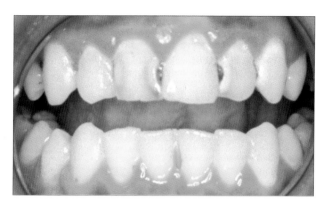

Fig. 1 Dental caries

The effect of dietary sugars

The fall in plaque pH when sugars enter the mouth and the subsequent recovery is called the *'Stephan curve'*

Inside the bacterial cells the sugars are converted by metabolic processes into organic acids as a waste product and excreted into the plaque fluid.

The acids accumulate in the plaque layer and cause demineralisation of the enamel surface.

SUGARS → PLAQUE → ACID → DEMINERALISATION

This 'acid attack' is more accurately described as a 'demineralisation episode' caused by the action of plaque bacteria on sugars entering the mouth.

Sucrose and glucose are the most important dietary sugars as they are added to many food products and beverages during manufacture. As table sugar, sucrose is often added during cooking or immediately before consumption. These simple sugars can enter the plaque bacteria and be metabolized within minutes of being consumed. Since plaque covers most tooth surfaces and reforms quickly after brushing, when acid forms within the plaque it acts almost like a layer of acid soaked blotting paper on the teeth.

Most people will consume some sugars as part of the everyday diet, but not everyone develops caries. To explain why this is so we must look in more detail at the factors that determine the risk from decay.

The pattern and severity of attack are determined by two groups of factors – those factors that influence the tooth's resistance to attack and those, in the environment of the tooth, which influence the severity of the attack.

THE TOOTH'S RESISTANCE

Largely because of their shape or position in the mouth some teeth are more resistant to attack than others. For example, in young people lower front teeth rarely decay because they do not have any grooves or fissures in which plaque can stagnate and they are bathed by saliva, which is beneficial. In contrast, the first permanent molar teeth have the highest decay rate because the deep fissures on the biting surfaces are difficult to clean.

In the UK neither malnutrition in the mother during pregnancy, nor in the child after birth, is likely to have any appreciable effect on the susceptibility of the teeth to decay. Calcium cannot be removed from the mother's teeth by the foetus during pregnancy or during lactation. The one factor that has been shown beyond doubt to reduce the rate of decay is fluoride and this is described below and in Section 2.

THE TOOTH'S ENVIRONMENT

The important factors within the mouth that interact to influence the severity of attack are plaque, dietary sugars, saliva and fluoride.

Sugars from the diet pass into the plaque within seconds of consumption. Many plaque bacteria use sugars as their source of energy and rapidly produce acid as a by-product. As acid is generated, it accumulates in the plaque layer and acidity in the plaque increases. Acidity is measured on the pH scale, and the lower the figure, the greater the degree of acidity. Figure 3 shows the effect of a sugar intake on plaque pH. The fall in plaque pH when sugars enter the mouth and the subsequent recovery as shown in the diagram is called the *'Stephan curve'*. This demineralization-remineralisation episode is sometimes referred to as an *'acid attack'*.

Within minutes of a sugar intake, sufficient acid may be generated within the absorbent plaque layer to cause a small outflow of calcium and phosphate from the enamel resulting in a tiny degree of demineralisation. After a period of time (usually about 20 minutes, but possibly up to 2 hours), the acid will have dissipated and the lost mineral may be slowly replaced from the saliva. This process is called *remineralisation*. However, if sugars are consumed frequently during the day, especially without the presence of other food or liquids that might dilute or help neutralise the acid, then the amount of demineralisation may outweigh remineralisation. This situation is illustrated in Figure 4a where a frequent intake of sugars during the day leads to an unfavourable proportion of total demineralisation to remineralisation periods, while an infrequent sugars intake results in a more favourable proportion as seen in Figure 4b.

If this imbalance persists over a period of time, then the gradual loss of mineral from the enamel may lead to its eventual breakdown and the formation of a cavity.

The type of bacteria that predominate within the plaque is influenced by the diet. Frequent consumption of sugars has been shown to

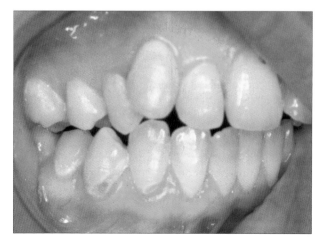

Fig. 2 Caries at the necks of teeth, from 'white spot' stage to cavitation

encourage the multiplication of bacteria that use sugars and can efficiently convert them to acid and it also increases the thickness of the plaque layer. The most commonly implicated plaque organism is *Strepococcus mutans,* however there are many other types that metabolise sugars to form acid. The proportion of these decay-causing bacteria falls when the amount and frequency of dietary sugars are reduced.

However, the mouth has its own defence mechanisms. While these are not fully understood, saliva is clearly the most important as it bathes the plaque on the tooth surface and helps to neutralise the acids and wash away sugars. This effect is enhanced if salivary flow after sugary snacks is stimulated for example by vegetables, cheese or sugar-free chewing gum. In addition, at the very earliest stages of the decay process, the tooth surface may 'heal' or 'remineralise' by deposition from saliva of calcium and phosphate, together with fluoride, which accelerates the healing process.

The early decay process may be seen as a contest fought at the tooth surface between the acids (resulting from the intake of sugars) causing demineralisation of the tooth surface and a number of factors including fluoride and saliva promoting the remineralisation of the tooth surface.

PREVENTION
There are two ways for individuals to reduce the risk of caries. The first is by using fluoride, easily and effectively done by brushing twice-daily with a fluoride toothpaste. The second is to reduce the severity of attack by decreasing the frequency and amount of consumption of sugars, the two being strongly linked. These methods will be discussed separately, but should be used together in order to improve or maintain oral health.

FLUORIDE
Fluoride toothpaste
The daily use of a fluoride toothpaste is a highly effective method of delivering fluoride to the tooth surface and has proved to be a major benefit. To some extent its use has removed the need for professionally applied fluoride agents, except in special circumstances. To increase the benefit from fluoride toothpaste, the mouth should not be rinsed with water from a cup after toothbrushing. The paste should be spat out and the mouth rinsed with a little water transferred on the brush if desired. Care should be taken to ensure that young children do not eat toothpaste and brushing should be supervised by parents for those under 7 years of age. It is advised that parents should finish off the brushing to ensure that it has been done effectively and that the biting surfaces of any newly erupted teeth are cleaned, as they can be easily missed. The use of only a small pea-sized amount of toothpaste (with just a tiny smear for babies) is recommended by both the dental profession and manufacturers for children

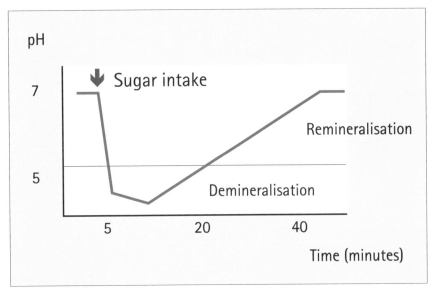

Fig. 3 The effect of sugar intake on plaque pH

under 7 years of age.[4] When fluoride drops or tablets are used, they should be given at a different time of day to brushing.

Water fluoridation
There are many natural sources of dietary fluoride, such as fish (bones) and tea and the drinking water supply in some areas. However, the most effective, safe and efficient public health measure for reducing dental caries is the fluoridation of public drinking water at a level of one part of fluoride per one million parts of water (1 ppm), which is equivalent to 1 mg F/litre. This is regarded as an optimum level. Since caries levels have fallen in many parts of the UK in the past 20 years, most experts now believe that water fluoridation should be targeted at areas where decay levels remain high.

Other fluoride agents
For extra protection against caries, fluoride gels and varnishes are effective and can be applied to the teeth by dentists, therapists and hygienists. For maximum benefit these should be applied every 3 or 4 months. Fluoride mouthrinses are also effective and are available for home use. These agents are of greatest value for the individuals who are most at risk to caries (*see* page 68).

Fluoride tablets and drops
Fluoride drops and tablets are available on prescription from dentists and doctors in the UK and may be purchased from pharmacists without a prescription. They were originally introduced to mimic the effect of water fluoridation by raising the dietary fluoride intake to what was considered to be an optimal level for caries control. For maximum effectiveness, daily administration from infancy until adolescence was required, although compliance with this regime was recognized as a frequent problem. Over the years the recommended dosage schedule has been reduced because of concerns that their use

Fluoride toothpaste

The daily use of a fluoride toothpaste is a highly effective method of delivering fluoride to the tooth surface

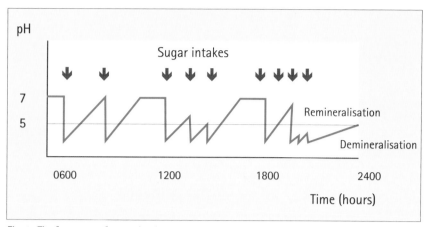

Fig. 4a The frequency of sugars intake

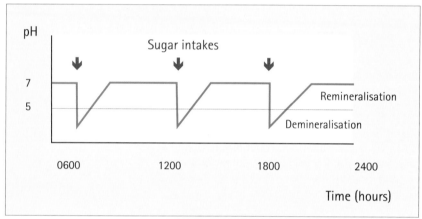

Fig. 4b Benefits of infrequent sugars intake

may be associated with a higher incidence of enamel fluorosis (*see* page 69). While initially seen as a potential public health measure, the introduction of fluoride toothpaste into the UK in the early 1970s has proved to be far more effective. Some experts now doubt the extent of any additional benefit that their use may provide beyond that achieved by effective twice-daily toothbrushing with a fluoride toothpaste. Today, their use should be confined to those at very high risk to caries or to those for whom dental treatment may be complicated by their general health (*see* page 68). Because of compliance problems, some clinicians prefer to rely on professionally applied topical fluoride agents such as fluoride varnishes or gels where additional measures are required. Fluoride drops or tablets should not be given in areas that have the optimum level of fluoride in the water supply and parents should therefore seek professional advice before use.

More information on fluoride is given in Section 2

DIET
Sugars in our diet
Food industry statistics estimate that almost half of the sucrose consumed by the public is sold as packaged sugar and about half is used by food, drink and confectionery manufacturers. The major industrial use of sucrose is the production of confectionery, which accounts for about a quarter of the total used in manufacturing, while the soft drinks industry uses about one fifth.

Nearly three-quarters of all sugars in the UK diet are added to foods during manufacture, cooking or before consumption. Confectionery, soft drinks, cakes, biscuits and table sugar (in tea and coffee, for example) are often consumed between meals and their frequent consumption is strongly linked to decay. The other sugars in the diet are naturally present in foods such as whole fruit, vegetables and milk. When sugars are consumed as part of these foods they are considered to be relatively unimportant as a cause of decay.

Dietary advice
Dietary advice should be aimed at changing the pattern of consumption of sugars with the aim of reducing the frequency and amount of consumption. The elimination of one or two sugar-sweetened items each day may be sufficient to enable remineralisation of the teeth to prevail over demineralisation, especially if fluoride from water or toothpaste is available. Food and drinks containing added sugars should be identified and limited, especially between meals. While fresh fruit and vegetables naturally contain sugars, their consumption is not linked to decay and they have an important place in our diet. Fruit juice and dried fruit can adversely affect teeth because of their high concentration of sugars and are not recommended for consumption between meals. Concentrated fruit juices should be well diluted with water. However, plain water is the safest drink as far as the teeth are concerned.

Parents and carers of infants should be warned of the dangers of putting fruit juice or sugars-sweetened drinks into feeding bottles, valve-type and reservoir feeders for the child to hold, especially in bed. Such practices result in almost continuous bathing of the enamel with sugars and lead to rapid tooth destruction. From six months of age, infants should be introduced to drinking from a cup. Free-flowing lidded feeding cups can help avoid spills in the early stages, before infants move on to an open beaker or cup. Feeding bottles should be discouraged after the age of 12 months.

People should also be encouraged to study the nutritional labels of food and drinks, and avoid frequently consuming those with high levels of sugars. The Food Standards Agency suggests a figure of 2 g of sugars per 100 g as a low sugar content, and 10 g per 100 g as a high content. Foods and drinks may contain added sugars other than sucrose. Glucose, maltose and fructose (when listed as an added sugar) are as likely to cause decay as sucrose and should not be used in infant health drinks and foods unless they are consumed only at mealtimes.

The use of sugars in medicines should also be strongly discouraged and sugar-free liquid medicines should be chosen by prescribers and when buying non-prescription medicines, whenever possible. If children have a long-term medical condition, parents and carers should request clinicians to prescribe sugar-free liquid medicines or preferably, tablets instead of liquids.

Preferable snacks and drinks for between-meal consumption

For between-meal snacks and drinks, raw vegetables such as carrots, fresh fruit, bread, low-fat unsweetened yoghurt, lower-fat cheese, skimmed or semi-skimmed milk and water can be recommended. Whole cow's milk should only be used as a main milk drink after the age of 1 year. Children between 1 and 2 years of age need whole milk. Between the ages of 2 and 5 years, provided they are eating a good varied diet, semi-skimmed milk can be introduced. Skimmed milk should not be given before the age of five. Milk and water are the only safe drinks for the teeth.

More information on diet and caries can be found in Section 3

PLAQUE CONTROL

Caries cannot develop without the presence of plaque, which is needed to convert dietary sugars into acid. Some research studies have shown that highly efficient toothbrushing techniques can reduce caries. But, plaque removal by normal tooth brushing alone does not appear to be as effective. Some plaque is left in fissures and other stagnation sites where caries occurs and plaque rapidly reforms on cleaned tooth surfaces. However brushing with a fluoride toothpaste combines plaque removal with the application of fluoride to the tooth surface and has proved to be highly effective.

Eating crisp or crunchy foods such as apples or raw carrots will not remove plaque effectively. However they are suitable snack foods and are an important part of a healthy diet.

More information on plaque control can be found in Section 5

FISSURE SEALANTS

A further way of helping to prevent dental caries is for a plastic film to be professionally applied to the pits and fissures of teeth as soon as possible after the teeth grow into the mouth. For the permanent molar teeth this is from the age of 6 years. The sealant prevents access of plaque and plaque acids to the enamel surface. Clinical trials have shown that sealants can be well retained and prevent caries. However, they are only effective on the biting surfaces of teeth. They are more cost effective in children at higher risk to caries and should be considered when there is a risk to general health from caries or dental treatment. In all cases fissure sealants should be seen as one part of a comprehensive preventive plan.

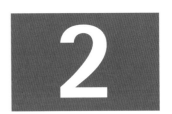

IN BRIEF
- Twice daily brushing with fluoride toothpaste is an effective preventive measure, but requires compliance. Evidence Base A
- A small pea-sized amount of fluoride toothpaste should be used by young children (a small smear for babies) and brushing with fluoride toothpaste should be supervised. Evidence Base C
- Water fluoridation is safe and effective, but should be targeted at communities with higher caries levels where it is technically feasible. Evidence Base A
- Fluoride supplements, though shown to be effective in clinical trials, may not be as effective in practice for home use or in community schemes. Evidence Base B

The scientific basis of oral health education. Part 2: Fluoride

R. S. Levine and C. R. Stillman-Lowe

FLUORIDE TOOTHPASTE

Fluoride toothpaste, which came into general use in the UK in the early 1970s, is now recognised as a development of the greatest importance to dental health. It is the most cost-effective topical fluoride agent for personal use and is thought to be the main reason for the decline in caries prevalence in Europe during the past 30 years. Fluoride toothpastes are currently available in three concentration ranges:

- Lower fluoride pastes containing less than 600 ppm,
- Standard pastes containing about 1000–1500 ppm,
- High concentration pastes containing over 2000 ppm.

The lower fluoride formulations were introduced to meet the concern that young children might ingest excessive fluoride. However, research has shown that the effectiveness of fluoride toothpastes increases with the fluoride concentration and there is no clear evidence that pastes containing less than 1000 ppm are effective. The use of lower concentration pastes may only be justified for children who are at low risk to caries, living in a fluoridated area, or receiving fluoride supplements. Indicators of low risk include little evidence of past caries activity and good oral hygiene suggesting regular use of fluoride toothpaste. Toothpastes containing 1000 to 1500 ppm are highly effective and should be used by all children from 7 years of age. Some toothpastes marketed as 'children's toothpaste' contain 1000 ppm but have a milder flavouring, to provide a more acceptable taste for children. The labelling of toothpastes remains unsatisfactory as the total fluoride content is not clearly marked in a simple form for the public to recognise.

While brands with similar fluoride concentrations may be equally effective, other components of the formulation may influence overall benefit. A number of leading brands have been independently evaluated in published long-term clinical trials in order to ensure efficacy. There is evidence that rinsing with water immediately after brushing with fluoride toothpaste reduces the benefit both in relation to the development of new cavities and the prevention of recurrent caries around fillings. It is preferable simply to spit out the paste and, if desired, the mouth rinsed with a little water transferred on the brush.

FLUORIDATION

Fluorides are compounds of the chemical element Fluorine. They are widely found in nature, in some foods such as fish (bones) in some plants such as tea, in beer and in some natural water supplies. The link between the presence of fluoride in public water supplies and reduced caries experience was first noticed early last century and has now been demonstrated by over 130 surveys in more than 20 countries including the UK. These surveys confirm that fluoride in the water at a concentration of about one part per million (1 ppm) reduces caries levels by up to half compared with similar non-fluoride areas. In 1945 Grand Rapids in the USA became the first community to have its water supply artificially adjusted to contain 1 ppm fluoride. Since then many cities around the world have followed, the largest schemes in the UK being in Birmingham, including parts of the West Midlands and Newcastle upon Tyne, where the improvement in children's dental health has been dramatic since fluoridation began.

The safety of water fluoridation is well docu-

Water fluoridation

In communities
where caries
prevalence remains
high, there are
significant potential
benefits to be gained
from fluoridation

mented. Numerous studies in both natural and artificially fluoridated areas have failed to show any adverse effect on general health at the level of 1 ppm, though fluoridation may be associated with an increase in dental fluorosis. One of the most authoritative reports is that of the Royal College of Physicians of England (1976). Fluoride's effectiveness and safety were upheld in the Court of Session judgment in Edinburgh in 1983.

Analysis of the reduction in treatment need after fluoridation has shown savings in manpower and resources. A large fall in the numbers of extractions and general anaesthetics administered to children has been reported. Furthermore, there is evidence from Scotland that the discontinuation of water fluoridation can result in a return to higher caries levels, despite the benefit of fluoride toothpaste. A 25% increase in caries prevalence was recorded 5 years after parts of Scotland were de-fluoridated. However, in some countries no change in caries levels has been seen after de-fluoridation. This might be caused by changes in diet or the increased use of fluoride toothpaste.

The evidence for the safety and benefits of fluoridation has led to support from the Committee on Child Health Services (1976), the Royal Commission of Inquiry into the Health Service (1979), the 1981 report of the Dental Strategy Review Group, The World Health Organisation (1998), the Independent Inquiry into Inequalities in Health (1998), the Medical Research Council (2002) and the All party Parliamentary Primary Care & Public Health Group (2003). This opinion has been embodied in guidance documents from the Department of Health, including *An Oral Health Strategy for England (1994), Modernising NHS Dentistry – Implementing the NHS Plan (2000),* and in England and Wales, the *Water Act 2004.*

A recent authoritative systematic review of 214 water fluoridation studies by the University of York found no clear evidence for a detrimental effect on general health.[5] The review concluded that the best available evidence suggests that fluoridation of the drinking water supply does reduce caries prevalence. However, it did conclude that the quality of many studies, which were done decades ago, did not meet today's rigorous research standards and that further research was needed to improve the evidence base on the safety and efficacy of water fluoridation.

While in some areas falling caries prevalence has reduced the absolute benefit to be gained from water fluoridation, in communities where prevalence remains high, often because of social and economic factors, there are significant potential benefits. Because of these changes, the consensus of expert opinion is that water fluoridation should be targeted at areas with higher caries levels.

FLUORIDE TABLETS AND DROPS

Supplementing the diet of children during the period of tooth development with fluoride in the form of tablets and drops is no longer considered to be an effective public health measure. Twice-daily toothbrushing with a fluoride toothpaste has proved to be highly effective and some experts believe that any additional benefit from the use of fluoride supplements may be small. Over the years the recommended dosage schedule has been reduced because of concerns that their use may be associated with a higher incidence of enamel fluorosis (*see* page 69).

Fluoride dietary supplements may be considered for those for whom the consequences of decay pose a hazard to general health or for whom dental treatment would be difficult because of their medical or physical condition. These groups include children with heart disease or cardiac defects who need pre-operative antibiotic cover for any dental procedure, as well as children prone to infection because of systemic disorders. Special needs children, those with mental or physical disabilities, may be more at risk to dental disease because of oral hygiene and dietary problems and may find dental treatment when needed, difficult or frightening. All of these children could benefit from fluoride supplements. The need for their use should be determined with dental advice and reviewed at intervals. Parents and carers should be advised of the benefits, and risks and especially of the long-term commitment, to the use of this measure, and of the importance of safe storage away from the reach of children.

The main problem with the use of fluoride dietary supplements is compliance with the required daily regime over the whole period of tooth formation. A stop-start pattern of use is unlikely to provide significant benefit. Some experts believe that compliance is likely to be higher in motivated families where the children may have a low risk of developing caries, while conversely, compliance may be poor in areas of social deprivation where the caries risk and the need for preventive measures is greater.

Fluoride supplements are licensed products and dosages appear in the British National Formulary/Dental Practitioners' Formulary as follows:

Daily dosage schedule for areas with less than 0.3 ppm F in the water supply:

6 months to 3 years — 0.25 mg F (0.5 mg NaF)

3 years up to 6 years — 0.5 mg F (1.1 mg NaF)

6 years and over — 1.0 mg F (2.2 mg NaF)

Once started, the continued need for fluoride supplements should be reviewed at intervals. It is generally advised that for maximum benefit their use be continued until the appearance of the second molar teeth, usually at about 11 to 12 years of age. However, this advice is based on the pre-eruptive effect of the ingested fluoride. Some experts believe that by allowing the tablets to dissolve slowly in the mouth a more beneficial topical post-eruptive effect may be achieved, both for older children and adults who may be at risk to caries.

For areas with 0.3 ppm or more F in the water

supply a lower dosage should be considered. While the schedule is provided for guidance, different dosages may be appropriate for individual patients and recommended dosages are periodically reviewed by expert groups.

In prescribing for individual patients, practitioners should determine the appropriate dosage schedule based on benefit, risk and compliance considerations and both the need and dosage should be reviewed at intervals. Fluoride supplements should be given daily, but the dose must not be increased if days are missed. No supplements should be given in areas where the water supply contains more than 0.7 ppm F. Local water companies and the Community Dental Service can confirm the fluoride content of the water supply.

FLUORIDATED MILK

The use of fluoridated milk for dental caries prevention was first proposed in the 1950s and school-based fluoridated milk programmes are now operating in 15 countries ranging from Russia to Chile. In the UK over 17,000 children in over 200 schools drink fluoridated milk at school as part of a programme that began in 1993 and was coordinated by the Liverpool Dental School. An additional potential benefit is that fluoridated milk may help displace sweetened soft drinks from the refrigerated vending machines found in many schools.

Results from early clinical trials indicate a reduction in caries levels comparable with those achieved by water fluoridation. However the organisation and maintenance of school-based programmes can pose problems where there is high absenteeism in infant and primary schools, or difficulty with the reliability of the milk distribution process.

ENAMEL FLUOROSIS

This much publicised condition presents as opaque or white areas, lines or flecks in the enamel surface and are most noticeable when they occur on front teeth. While these opacities can be due to a number of causes, one is the ingestion of excessive fluoride during the period of enamel formation. For incisor teeth the period of greatest risk is between 15 and 30 months of age. The more severe cosmetically unacceptable forms are uncommon in the UK, but may result from the use of fluoride dietary supplements in optimally fluoridated areas or from the eating of fluoride toothpaste in early childhood. The use of fluoride toothpaste in areas with optimally fluoridated water supplies has been shown by surveys using sensitive photographic recording to result in only a small increase in the mildest forms, which mostly pass unnoticed. No increase in moderate or severe forms has yet been detected, and simple techniques are available to improve the appearance of affected teeth. Nevertheless, this is an area of concern to both the public and the dental professions and care should be taken to ensure that young children do not ingest excessive amounts of fluoride toothpaste, especially in fluoridated areas or when fluoride supplements are used. While manufacturers rightly endeavour to make the taste of children's toothpaste attractive, there is concern that the use of food flavouring such as strawberry may encourage excessive consumption.

To reduce the risk of fluorosis, parents should supervise toothbrushing of children under 7 years of age and should place an amount of toothpaste no greater than the size of a small pea on the brush (or a small smear for babies). Brushing should be done normally no more than twice each day and the child should be encouraged to spit out afterwards, rather than rinse with water. Supervision will continue to be beneficial beyond this age. When fluoride drops or tablets are used, they should be given at a different time of day to brushing.

HOW DOES FLUORIDE WORK?

Teeth and bone are composed largely of a crystalline mineral compound of calcium and phosphate called *hydroxyapatite*. Research over the past 60 years has shown that fluoride produces its effect in a number of different ways which combine to slow and help prevent the decay process and also to reverse decay in its early stages. These are given below in the order of effectiveness.

- *Enhanced remineralisation* – Very low levels of fluoride in the plaque and saliva are able to alter the chemical balance between demineralisation of the enamel and remineralisation. The effect favours the remineralisation process, allowing the early carious attack on enamel to be reversed and new mineral crystals, with better structure and greater acid resistance, to be deposited. This is the mechanism by which fluoride toothpaste is thought to work and appears to be the most important.
- *Reduced acid production* – Fluoride is concentrated in the plaque layer on the surfaces of the teeth and reduces the conversion of dietary sugars into acid by plaque bacteria. Fluoride toothpaste also invokes this mechanism.
- *Fluoride substitution* – Fluoride entering the developing teeth from the diet via the blood stream is incorporated into the new mineral crystals. The partly fluoridated hydroxyapatite that is formed is theoretically more resistant to acid attack than that formed without fluoride.
- *Reduced pit and fissure depth* – The parts of the teeth most susceptible to caries are the natural pits and grooves, or fissures on the biting surfaces of back teeth. Fluoride entering the developing teeth at an early stage appears to result in reduced pit and fissure depth.

The use of fluoride toothpaste, which delivers its effect at the tooth surface, has reduced the significance of the last two mechanisms, which are now thought to play a very minor role.

Fluorosis

To reduce the risk of fluorosis, parents should supervise toothbrushing for children under seven years of age, and use a small pea-sized blob of paste

IN BRIEF

- The frequency and amount of consumption of sugars in drinks and foods are the most important risk factors. Evidence Base A
- Sugars-sweetened snacks and drinks should be avoided between meals and especially at bedtime. Evidence Base B
- Naturally occurring sugars when consumed in fresh whole fruit, vegetables and cereal grains are not a risk factor for dental caries and these items are an essential part of a health balanced diet. Evidence Base B

The scientific basis of oral health education. Part 3: Diet and oral health

R. S. Levine and C. R. Stillman-Lowe

SUGARS AND DENTAL CARIES

The evidence for a link between sugars and caries comes from a variety of sources. Epidemiological studies have shown a clear correlation between caries experience and mean sugars consumption levels in different countries. When communities have shown changes in sugars consumption, such as during World War II (1939–1945) when consumption fell, a corresponding fall in caries prevalence has been observed. Similarly, groups having low or restricted sugars consumption and those with high consumption of sugars, show corresponding lower or higher levels of caries experience. Children using sugars-sweetened medicines over long periods have shown higher caries levels compared with a control group. Human clinical studies have demonstrated that, when sugars consumption is increased under controlled conditions, then the caries increment follows and it falls when consumption is reduced. Laboratory studies have shown, by the use of miniature pH electrodes inserted into the plaque on teeth, an immediate fall in pH on the application of a neutral sugar solution, with the acidity persisting for 20 minutes to 2 hours.

SUGARS IN FOOD AND DRINKS

The sugars most responsible for dental caries have been classified by the Committee on Medical Aspects of Food Policy (now the Scientific Advisory committee on Nutrition) as *non-milk extrinsic sugars* (NMES),[6] as shown in Figure 1.

NMES are those which are added to food and drinks during processing, manufacture or preparation. NMES also include sugars naturally present in fresh fruit juices, honey and syrups. The reason that NMES are implicated is that they are simple sugars that can rapidly enter the plaque

bacteria and be converted to acid and are often frequently consumed in amounts far in excess of nutritional needs. Sugars naturally present in fruit and vegetables – and eaten as such – are not considered to be cariogenic. This is because they are contained within the cell structure of the plant and may not be fully released into the mouth during eating. Fruit and vegetables are an essential part of a health diet. Concentrated fruit juices and dried fruits have a high concentration of sugars. While these are included within the fruit and vegetables recommended by the '5 a day' programme, sponsored by the Department of Health in England, from a dental perspective their frequent consumption especially between meals could increase the risk of caries. It should be noted that fresh fruit juices and dried fruit, irrespective of how much is consumed, may each only constitute one of the five daily portions and this point should be stressed when giving dietary advice. Lactose, the sugar in milk, is less cariogenic than other dietary sugars. When naturally present in milk, it appears to be virtually non-cariogenic.

The common non-milk extrinsic dietary sugars are sucrose (refined from beet and cane), glucose, maltose (extracted from many foods) and fructose (extracted from fruit). Fructose is also a NMES when naturally present in natural unsweetened fruit juice, honey and syrups and when used as an additive to foods and drinks. Significant amounts of glucose and fructose are now made industrially from starch. While sucrose is highly cariogenic, animal studies have shown that both glucose and fructose will readily produce caries and combinations of these sugars appear to be as cariogenic as sucrose alone.

Furthermore, there does not appear to be a safe level for sugars concentration in food and

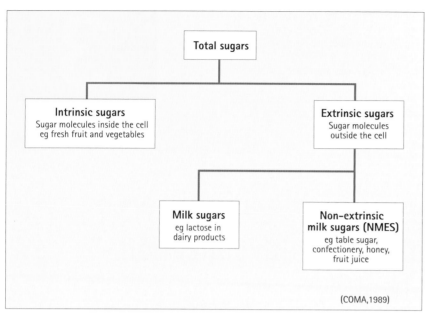

Fig. 1 Classification of sugars

Cariogenic sugars
These sugars are described in Tables 1 and 2.

Non-cariogenic sweeteners
These can be classed as either bulk or intense sweeteners (Table 3).

Table 3 Bulk sweeteners mainly used to add sweetness, calories and bulk to confectionery products

Maltitol syrup	Lactitol
Mannitol	Xylitol
Isomalt	Maltitol
Sorbitol	

Xylitol
There is considerable evidence from laboratory and clinical studies that xylitol is not only non-cariogenic, but also suppresses the growth of acidogenic bacteria in plaque. There is additional evidence that beneficial effect on the plaque bacteria may be passed from a mother to her children. The use of xylitol in chewing gum has been the subject of a number of extensive clinical trials, which generally have shown a significant caries-inhibiting effect. Xylitol-sweetened chewing gum may provide a benefit for caries prevention.[7]

If consumed in excess, bulk sweeteners can have a laxative effect. While overt diarrhoea is a rare side effect, children are at greater risk. There is a statutory requirement for these sweeteners to carry the labelling excessive consumption may produce laxative effects.

Table 4 lists intense sweeteners added in small amounts, often to soft drinks.

Table 4 Intense sweeteners added in small amounts, often to soft drinks

Acesulfame K	Aspartame
Saccharin	Cyclamate
Thaumatin	Sucralose
Neohesperidine DC	

Combinations of sugars and intense sweeteners such as saccharin are used in some products; however the latter will not have a protective role and such products must be classified as cariogenic. Concentrated soft drinks, which are the main source of artificial sweeteners in the diet of young children, should be diluted with extra water for these young consumers to avoid excessive intake. Even if well diluted, such drinks are acidic and have the potential to cause erosion.

It must be remembered that manufacturing problems related to sugars substitution are not just limited to sweetness, cost and safety. Sugars give bulk to many foods and influence properties such as viscosity, texture, and shelf life.

The pattern of sugar intake
After consuming sugar, acid is rapidly generated

drinks, as this is linked in a complex manner with physical consistency. Indeed, in solution, sucrose concentrations below the taste threshold can generate acid in plaque.

Dietary starch, which is a complex carbohydrate, is converted to maltose and glucose in the mouth by enzymes in saliva, and these sugars are then available for metabolizing into acids by plaque bacteria. However, the rate of conversion is slow and dietary starch by itself is very much less important than dietary sugars as a cause of dental caries. Recent research has shown that when starch is cooked at very high temperatures, such as for the production of some snack foods, then the conversion to glucose in the mouth can occur more rapidly.

From a theoretical aspect, sugar-free chewing gum may have a positive benefit for dental health by increasing salivary flow during chewing, which helps to neutralise plaque acid activity. The majority of clinical studies have found a positive benefit.

Table 1 Sugars and other compounds added to food and drinks during processing, manufacture or before consumption as sweeteners and that have the potential to cause dental caries

Glucose*	Maltose
Fructose*	Glucose syrup
Hydrolysed starch	Maltodextrins
Sucrose*	Oligofructose

*Non-cariogenic when contained in whole fresh fruits, vegetables and grains.

Table 2 Products which are essentially a mixture of sugars

Brown sugar (mainly sucrose)	Treacle
Maple syrup	Honey
Golden syrup	

in the dental plaque and, within 1-2 minutes, plaque pH has fallen to levels that favour enamel demineralisation. The return to neutrality takes between 20 minutes and 2 hours, depending on such factors as salivary flow rate and buffering capacity and plaque thickness and composition. Maximum acid production is achieved by modest sugar concentrations, beyond which increased concentrations do not give a greater fall in pH. However, frequent sugar intakes will not allow time for the pH to recover and will prolong the period of plaque acidity. This pattern may allow demineralisation to exceed remineralisation resulting in a progressive loss of minerals from enamel as shown in Figure 4a (*see* page 64).

These observations are supported by animal experiments that have shown a direct correlation between sucrose frequency and caries levels.

It has been shown that, in human volunteers who stopped toothbrushing and used 2-hourly sucrose rinses, enamel demineralisation occurred within 3 weeks. However, as the amount of NMES consumed has been shown to be independently related to caries experience and as frequency and amount are strongly linked, advice must be to reduce both. This advice is supported by a report from the Committee on Medical Aspects of Food Policy (*Dietary Sugars and Human Disease 1989*).[6]

The frequency and time of consumption of sugars-sweetened foods and drinks have both been shown to be important factors in determining caries levels. Sugars consumed with main meals appear to be of less significance because they are cleared from the mouth by other foods and the high salivary flow rate generated by eating. Other foods taken as part of the meal, such as cheese may help stimulate salivary flow and raise the calcium level in plaque so that remineralisation is promoted. However, the same sugars-sweetened items consumed between meals appear to have a much more detrimental effect as well as increasing the total daily frequency count.

Recent research has confirmed that bedtime is the worst time to consume a sugars-sweetened drink or snack. This is caused by the low salivary flow rate during sleep and to the fact that toothbrushing is unlikely to remove all traces of any sugary snack taken before bed. Children who consumed both a sugary drink and snack in the hour before bed were found to have four times the number of decayed teeth compared with children who had neither.[8]

Sugars in medicines can also cause decay. Many paediatric medicines, including those sold without prescription, have sugar-free alternatives. Clinicians should prescribe sugar-free medicines and parents/carers should request them. Pharmacists should be encouraged to stock and recommend sugar-free alternatives to the most commonly used prescription and general sale medicines.

Caries levels

The frequency and time of consumption of sugars-sweetened foods and drinks are important factors in determining caries levels

IN BRIEF
- The risk of developing periodontal disease can be reduced by careful and effective daily toothbrushing. **Evidence Base A**
- The risk of developing periodontal disease can be reduced by not smoking. **Evidence Base B**

The scientific basis of oral health education.
Part 4: Periodontal diseases

R. S. Levine and C. R. Stillman-Lowe

While there are a number of diseases, both acute and chronic, that affect the gums and the surrounding bone and fibres that support the teeth, by far the most common are gingivitis and chronic periodontitis. Gingivitis can begin as early as childhood and presents as inflammation of the gum margin, with redness, swelling and bleeding on brushing (Fig. 1). Most forms of gingivitis can be reversed by effective oral hygiene. Without adequate personal oral care, a second stage, termed chronic periodontitis can occur. In this stage, which can begin as early as adolescence, the bone and fibres that support the teeth are progressively destroyed (Fig. 2). However, the rate of destruction can vary greatly both between and within individuals. This may lead eventually to loosening and finally loss of the tooth, although the process can be slowed by a combination of personal care and professional treatment.

CAUSE

Periodontal diseases are caused by dental plaque – a soft, sticky film composed mainly of bacteria, which forms on the teeth and is present in all mouths. Bacterial plaque causes a complex response in the individual that the body intends to be protective. However, if the body's immunological defence system is not functioning properly, then damage to the periodontal tissues can occur. Similarly, if the amount or virulence of the bacteria increases, then the body's response may not be sufficient to prevent damage. The severity of the damage caused by plaque is determined by a number of factors that fall into two groups – those that cause plaque to be retained on the teeth, and those that modify the nature of the tissue reaction to the bacterial products. The overall balance between the bacte-

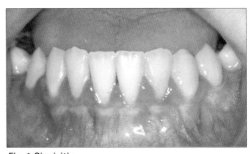

Fig. 1 Gingivitis

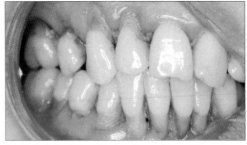

Fig. 2 Periodontitis, with abrasion cavities at the necks of teeth caused by incorrect toothbrushing technique

rial challenge and the body's response is critical to the maintenance of periodontal health – an upset to the balance (on either side) can result in the development and progression of periodontal disease.

Plaque retention factors

Any irregularity around the teeth will encourage the accumulation of plaque by making tooth cleaning difficult. Such factors include crooked teeth, overhanging edges on fillings, poorly contoured fillings, some types of partial dentures, and calculus. Calculus (tartar) is plaque which has become calcified and hardened and may

Prevention of periodontal disease

The main way of limiting periodontal disease is by plaque control directed to maintaining gingival health

cause plaque stagnation. Calculus can form above the gum line (supragingival) and below the gum margin (subgingival). As periodontal disease progresses, the shallow space between the gum margin and the tooth deepens to form a periodontal pocket in which plaque and subgingival calculus accumulate.

Modifying factors

There is a strong association between the amount of plaque accumulation and the reaction of the oral tissues. However, variations are seen both in the reaction of the gums and the rate of destruction of the supporting bone. This may be caused by a number of factors. The types of bacteria present in plaque vary both between individuals and at different sites within an individual mouth. There is considerable evidence that smoking increases the risk of periodontal disease and reduces the effectiveness of treatment. In many cases, however, the cause of variation is likely to be differences between individuals in the susceptibility of their tooth-supporting structures to the destructive processes caused by bacterial products.

The gum margin around the necks of the teeth is a unique structure in the body as it is an imperfect junction between two quite different body tissues; hard, calcified tooth surface and the soft, vascular tissue of the gums. The body's immunological defence system has to fight a constant battle to prevent harmful bacteria from penetrating this junction and anything that affects this defence system can produce a reaction at the gum margin, usually inflammation. This was first seen as scurvy in seamen before the need for vitamin C was recognised. However today, a common example is the change produced by the hormonal disturbance during pregnancy, where even modest deposits of plaque can produce a condition known as pregnancy gingivitis. Other systemic conditions that can cause gingival change, often as a first indication, include anaemia, diabetes, HIV/AIDS and leukaemia.

PREVENTION

As gingivitis precedes adult periodontitis, the main way of limiting periodontal disease is by plaque control directed to maintaining gingival health. This must be considered at two levels – what people can do for themselves by way of plaque control on a daily basis, and what dentists and hygienists/therapists can do to eliminate plaque retention factors and to advise the individual on the most appropriate home care.

What people can do for themselves

The most important plaque control method is effective tooth brushing with a fluoride toothpaste and it should be established as a daily routine from the time of tooth eruption. Tooth brushing skills should be taught to people of all ages. The precise technique is less important than the result, which is that plaque is removed effectively and daily without causing damage to the teeth or gums.

A gentle scrub technique is effective for most people and is easy to teach and readily accepted. Careful use of this method with a recommended type of brush should be encouraged as it will provide effective plaque removal. Most authorities recommend a brush with a small head bearing densely packed soft to medium synthetic filaments. Faulty tooth brushing techniques involving excessive pressure may considerably increase gum recession and loss of tooth substance by mechanical abrasion and must therefore be corrected (Fig. 2).

Plaque disclosing agents which colour plaque to make it easily visible can be a useful aid to improving plaque control. They will not in themselves remove plaque, but will show areas where plaque remains after brushing. Dental floss and other interdental cleaning aids are of value if used correctly but they will usually require professional advice and instruction. An additional method of plaque control is the use of antiseptics, of which chlorhexidine is the most effective. Although this antiseptic is on general sale in the UK in mouthrinse and gel forms, its tendency to stain teeth and impair taste makes it generally unacceptable for long-term use. Many popular toothpastes contain other chemical plaque suppressing agents such as triclosan combined with a copolymer or zinc salts. While these are less effective than chlorhexidine, they do not have the same side-effects and have been shown to be of value to gingival health.

What dental professionals can do

It is the responsibility of the dentist to ensure that any treatment provided minimises plaque retention; this is a part of treatment planning. Clear advice must be given on the need to clean bridges, dentures and orthodontic appliances (braces) effectively and regularly. Calculus that forms on the teeth above the gum level and within the pockets should be removed regularly by careful professional scaling. While appropriate professional treatment is important, the highest priority should be given to effective daily oral hygiene by the individual.

More information on plaque control can be found in Section 5.

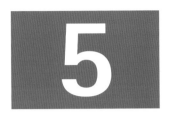

The scientific basis of oral health education. Part 5: Plaque control and dental diseases

R. S. Levine and C. R. Stillman-Lowe

There is ample evidence of an association between plaque and periodontal disease in children and adults. Plaque deposits have been shown to cause gingival inflammation, which is reversed by plaque removal. It follows that plaque control can be endorsed for the prevention of gingivitis, although it should be remembered that once the bone and fibres supporting the tooth have been lost as a result of chronic periodontitis, then plaque control alone is probably insufficient to stabilise the condition. A combination of personal plaque control and professional treatment may then be needed to retard further bone loss.

Based on clinical observation, it had been suggested that dental caries could be controlled by highly effective toothbrushing, without the benefit of fluoride toothpaste. Some research studies have shown that highly efficient toothbrushing techniques can reduce caries. However, plaque removal by normal toothbrushing alone does not appear to be as effective, as some plaque is left in fissures and other stagnation sites where caries occurs, and plaque rapidly begins to reform on cleaned tooth surfaces. For caries prevention, the real value of toothbrushing is now thought to be that it combines plaque removal with the application of fluoride to the tooth surface.

PLAQUE REMOVAL FOR CHILDREN

It is generally agreed that most children have insufficient manual dexterity to achieve effective plaque removal with a toothbrush until at least 6 to 7 years of age. Parents should be advised to brush their children's teeth thoroughly twice a day using a small brush. One method of toothbrushing is for the parent to stand behind the child and tilt the child's head upwards so that all tooth surfaces can be brushed using a gentle scrub motion.

PLAQUE REMOVAL FOR ADULTS

The gentle scrub method of toothbrushing is effective in plaque removal and is easily taught and accepted. It should be carried out with a small toothbrush for ease of access. The method is to place the filaments of the brush at the neck of the tooth and to use very short horizontal movements to dislodge plaque from the stagnation areas at the gum margins around the teeth. The biting surfaces of side and back teeth should then be brushed. Emphasis should be placed on small movements and gentle pressure, together with an unhurried systematic approach to the cleaning of all surfaces. Holding the brush with the fingers in a 'pen' grip may avoid excessive force.

The use of dental floss, mini-brushes and similar interdental cleaning aids can be of great value in individual cases, but specific professional advice and guidance is necessary and care must be taken to avoid damaging the gums. Such aids should be used as an addition to toothbrushing and must not be considered as an alternative.

RECOMMENDED TOOTHBRUSH SPECIFICATIONS

While there is a wide variation in toothbrush design, little evidence exists to support specific recommendations. The size of the toothbrush head should be appropriate to the user but it should be remembered that a smaller head will give better access to the back of the mouth and those tooth surfaces that a large headed brush cannot reach. The filaments (bristles) should be of a synthetic material, round-ended and of a soft to medium texture. For children or adults

Toothbrush replacement

When the bristles become deformed or splayed, plaque removal becomes less effective and the toothbrush should be replaced

with limited manual dexterity, it can be an advantage to choose a toothbrush with a large handle that provides a firm, comfortable grip. When the bristles become deformed or splayed, plaque removal becomes less effective and the toothbrush should be replaced.

POWERED TOOTHBRUSHES

Modern powered toothbrushes have become very popular. An independent systematic review of existing studies concluded that powered toothbrushes are at least as effective as manual toothbrushes and there is no evidence that they will cause more injuries to the gums than manual brushes.[9] Powered toothbrushes with a rotation oscillation action (ie the head rotates in one direction and then the other) have been shown to be slightly better at removing plaque and reducing gum inflammation than manual toothbrushes, but the long-term benefits are unclear. Some individuals like the 'feel' of powered toothbrushes and they can be helpful in those with limited manual dexterity, such as arthritis sufferers; furthermore, the novelty value in children can encourage compliance with their brushing regime. As with manual toothbrushes, the heads do wear out and need to be replaced regularly.

CHEMICAL PLAQUE SUPPRESSANTS

Of the many agents that have been tested, chlorhexidine has proved to be the most effective plaque suppressant under clinical conditions. It is on general sale in the UK in mouthrinse, gel and spray forms and is used in the management of periodontal disease. It can cause staining of teeth, which is difficult to remove from white fillings and can impair taste. While clinical experience in daily sustained use is limited, 2 years being the duration of the longest clinical trial reported to date, no other major adverse effects have been reported. Nevertheless, it is generally unacceptable for long-term unsupervised use, 1 month being the normal limit. It can be of value for short-term use when toothbrushing is difficult or painful, but works best on clean teeth by inhibiting plaque formation.

Other antiseptics without the adverse effects of chlorhexidine are used in many mouthrinses and toothpastes. One of the more effective of these appears to be the phenol derivative, triclosan, when combined with a co-polymer or with zinc compounds. Use of such products may provide benefits to plaque control and gingival health. There is evidence that the non-cariogenic sweetener xylitol inhibits the growth of some plaque bacteria (*see* Page 72). However, its value for the prevention of periodontal disease has not been established.

6

The scientific basis of oral health education. Part 6: Erosion

R. S. Levine and C. R. Stillman-Lowe

Erosion is the loss of tooth substance caused by the direct action of chemicals on the tooth surface. It is quite different from caries in both appearance and causation. While erosion can occur by chemical action alone, it is sometimes linked to attrition of the teeth due to grinding them, often at night, or eating coarse foods and with abrasion caused by excessive brushing with a hard brush or an abrasive toothpaste. Erosion is therefore classed as a type of tooth wear. Indeed, tooth wear in many individuals is caused by a combination of attrition, abrasion and erosion in differing proportions.

CLINICAL PRESENTATION

Erosion was described as early as 1892 among Sicilian lemon pickers. The characteristic appearance is loss of enamel and in more severe cases of dentine from specific sites. Erosion should not be confused with caries. While caries affects the surfaces of the teeth where plaque stagnates, erosion affects plaque-free surfaces. Primarily, these are the palatal (inside) aspects of the upper front teeth followed by the labial (lip) aspects of these teeth and the occlusal (biting) surfaces of the premolar (side) and molar (back) teeth (Fig. 1). In the deciduous dentition the incisal (biting) edges of the upper front teeth are often lost first (Fig. 2).

In the early stages pain is not a feature, but as enamel loss progresses, sensitivity to thermal change and acidic drinks becomes established and more persistent pain can occur in severe cases.

CAUSE

Erosion is usually caused by acids entering the mouth. However cases have been reported amongst workers in the chemical industry and

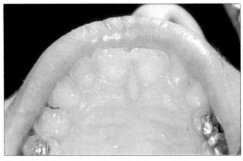

Fig. 1 Dental erosion on the palatal aspect of upper anterior teeth. Almost all of the enamel has been lost

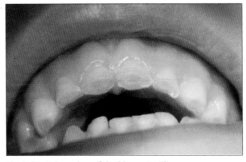

Fig. 2 Dental erosion of deciduous teeth

acid battery factories due to atmospheric fumes and from careless use of pipettes in laboratories.

While industrial cases appear to have diminished because of increased awareness in the workplace, two other causes may have become more important. Gastric reflux brings acid into the mouth and is thought to affect up to 70% of individuals at some time. Causes include hiatus hernia, pregnancy, motion sickness, alcoholism, obesity and bulimia, of which it can be an early sign. However, dietary factors are thought to be the most common cause today. While citrus

Fruit and tooth erosion

Fruit juice is erosive, but there is little evidence to link the consumption of whole fruit with increased erosion in a normal population

fruits have erosive potential, there is little evidence to link the consumption of whole fruit with increased erosion in a normal population.

In contrast, fruit juice is erosive and the frequent consumption of juices has been linked in many reports to increased tooth wear, as have sports-type drinks. Possibly of greater significance is the erosive potential of soft drinks, including carbonated and fruit based ones. The rapid rise in consumption of fruit juice and soft drinks, following the development of modern containers such as the tetrapak, plastic bottles and aluminium cans, has been blamed for what is generally perceived as an increase in the prevalence of erosion, especially among youngsters. The relationship between frequency of consumption of such drinks and erosion is now established.

The principal ingredient linked to erosion is citric acid, which is found in most fruit juices and soft drinks, however other fruit acids may have an effect. The erosive effect is partly caused by its low pH and also because it can demineralise enamel by binding to calcium and removing it from the tooth surface, a process called chelation. Cola-type drinks may also contain phosphoric acid, which produces a low pH. The recent popularity of 'alcopop' type drinks, which are fruit-flavoured alcoholic beverages and strong ciders, all of which have a low pH, has caused concern, but as yet no substantive evidence is available. While the pH of a drink is an indicator of its erosive potential, a measure called total titratable acidity, which gives the capacity of a liquid to dissolve mineral, is a better guide.

However, some other factors are important in determining the risk of erosion. These include the flow rate and buffering capacity of saliva, the manner and frequency of consumption of erosive drinks and the consumption of other foods such as cheese and milk. There is anecdotal evidence that the common habit of swishing carbonated drinks around the mouth before swallowing may increase the danger. In addition, acidic ice lollipops and acid-based sweets may have erosive potential.

At present we lack a universally accepted index for the assessment of erosion and consequently no reliable long-term data to indicate changes in the prevalence of erosion over time. However, most clinicians believe that prevalence has increased during the past 20 years. From the many studies in the literature the prevalence of enamel erosion in children appears to vary from less than 10% to 50% according to age For erosion into dentine the figures are lower, but may affect 25% children with deciduous teeth. These figures are supported by the 1993 *National Child Dental Health Survey.*[10] The higher levels usually found in the deciduous dentition are thought to be due to the practice of giving fruit juice in feeding bottles or feeder cups.

PREVENTION

Erosion can be prevented by reducing the intake of erosive drinks and food. While no safe limit can be established any reduction is desirable. Children and young adults especially, should not have acidic beverages as their main fluid intake. The practices of swishing and frequent sipping of acidic drinks should be discouraged. Taking milk or cheese afterwards may be beneficial. Drinking erosive beverages through a straw has been shown to help, but only if the tip is placed well back in the mouth. It is also sensible to avoid tooth brushing for a period of time after an erosive episode as the brush can damage the softened enamel. There is no conclusive evidence as to how long this should be, but a period of 1 hour is accepted by most experts.

The resistance of the teeth to erosion can be increased by the use of topical fluorides. Whilst twice daily use of a fluoride toothpaste is considered essential, mouthrinses are also of value. The professional application of fluoride varnishes and gels can give added benefit, both by increasing enamel acid resistance and in reducing sensitivity. In severe cases some form of restoration is usually necessary, often crowns for permanent teeth.

Where gastric regurgitation is suspected because of physical or emotional problems such as bulimia, the patient should be advised to consult their medical practitioner.

The scientific basis of oral health education. Part 7: Oral cancer

R. S. Levine and C. R. Stillman-Lowe

ORAL TUMOURS

As elsewhere in the body, both benign and malignant tumours can occur in the mouth. Benign tumours tend to be slow growing and localized and are rarely life-threatening. However, malignant tumours can grow rapidly, infiltrate the surrounding area and spread to the lymph glands and other parts of the body, with the formation of secondary or metastatic deposits, especially in the bones, lungs or other organs. If detected early and treated, a complete cure is often possible, but delay makes treatment difficult and approximately half of all cases prove fatal within 5 years.

SQUAMOUS CELL CARCINOMA

The most common type of oral cancer is squamous cell carcinoma which accounts for about 90% of all oral malignancies. They arise from the oral mucosa lining the mouth and covering the tongue. In the majority of cases they present as an ulcer, most commonly in the floor of the mouth, the lateral border of the tongue, or

inside the lips. Often they arise within a pre-existing white, red or thickened area of mucosa and at the earliest stage may not show obvious signs of ulceration. Thickened white areas of mucosa, termed leukoplakia, are well recognized as potential sites for malignant change and the appearance of red spots or ulceration within a leukoplakia is often an indication of this change (Fig. 1). Malignant ulcers differ from other innocent ulcers by persisting for more than 2 weeks after any cause is removed. Unlike other forms of oral ulceration, they do not heal or resolve spontaneously. Indeed, any ulcer present for more than 3 weeks should be investigated without delay.

OTHER ORAL TUMOURS

Other tumours can arise in or around the mouth, such as within the jaw bones or from salivary glands, connective tissue, blood vessels or nerves. These tumours generally present as swellings, but in some cases the first signs may be loosening of teeth, spontaneous fracture of the jaw or enlargement of the lymph glands in the neck.

PREVALENCE AND PROGNOSIS

It is estimated that there are about 4,500 new cases of oral cancer each year in the UK, with more than 2,000 deaths. The number of cases is increasing and approaches that for cervical cancer, but the overall 5-year survival rate is worse and the mortality rate is higher than for most other cancers. For oral cancers detected at the earliest stage the 5-year survival rate is about 90%, but this falls to about 20% for those presenting at the latest stage. The poor overall 5-year survival rate is thought to due to the late

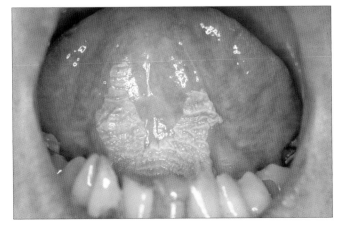

Fig. 1
Leukoplakia on the ventral (surface) of the tongue

Oral cancer

The main risk factors are tobacco or alcohol and a combination of these factors appears to multiply the risk

presentation of many cases. This finding is even more distressing because the mouth is the easiest body cavity to examine. While most cases occur in men, and many cases occur in the over 60s, in recent years there has been a shift towards an earlier age of onset (45–59 years) and an increase in the number of women affected.[11]

CAUSE AND PREVENTION

The main risk factors for oral cancer are tobacco or alcohol and a combination of these factors appears to multiply the risk. The relative risk for long-term smokers who also consume alcohol may be over 30 times greater than non-smokers who are infrequent drinkers. The habits of chewing tobacco and reverse smoking (with the lit end inside the mouth) have been found to be factors, while the common practice amongst some Asian communities of chewing 'betel nut quid', 'paan' or 'ghutka', an addictive blend of tobacco and other vegetable matter, is linked to the high prevalence of oral cancer in the Indian sub-continent and Asian communities in other parts of the world. There is evidence that if smoking ceases then the risk of developing oral cancer falls and about 50% of leukoplakias appear to resolve. Other risk factors include pre-existing white patches on the oral mucosa, including those related to candida infection *(see next section),* some viral infections and immuno-suppressive conditions such as AIDS/HIV.

There is evidence that the prevention of many types of malignancy benefit from a higher intake of fresh fruit and vegetables, resulting from their content of vitamin and anti-oxidant compounds. In all cases early diagnosis is vital and argues the case for regular whole mouth examinations and immediate referral of suspicious lesions to an appropriate secondary care clinician.

The scientific basis of oral health education. Part 8: Other oral diseases

R. S. Levine and C. R. Stillman-Lowe

There are a number of other conditions that can develop in the mouth and require professional advice and help.

ORAL CANDIDOSIS

Infection with the fungus *Candida albicans* can present in the mouth in many forms, both acute and chronic. The most common presentations are **angular chelitis**, a chronic infection of the angles of the mouth, usually seen in older people, especially those with old, worn dentures (Fig. 1) and **denture sore mouth** a chronic infection usually seen in the palate where a denture is worn at night, instead of being removed as generally advised (Fig. 2). Some cases are associated with poor nutrition, chronic anaemia, diabetes or depression of the immune system as in AIDS/HIV infection. Prevention of these common forms depends on treating any systemic factors and the removal and thorough cleaning of dentures each night and replacement when they are worn out (*see* Section 10).

ORAL ULCERATION

About 25% of the population suffers from **minor apthous ulceration** – the common mouth ulcer – on a regular basis. The ulcers occur either singly or in small crops, often inside the lips or cheek and heal with or without treatment within 10 days. The cause remains unknown, although some cases are associated with systemic illness such as anaemia or diabetes. A more severe form, **major apthous ulceration,** generally produces solitary ulcers, which take up to a month to heal, often leaving a residual scar.

Herpes simplex infection can cause a common form of oral ulceration. Viral in origin, it can produce a very sore mouth with crops of small grey ulcers, that generally heal sponta-

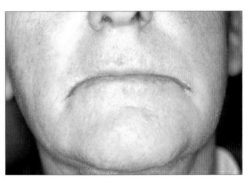

Fig. 1 Angular chelitis, a form of chronic candida infection

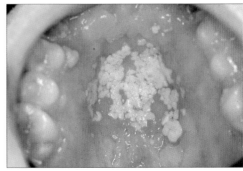

Fig. 2 Candida infection in the palate associated with poor hygiene practice in the wearing of a partial upper denture. The yellow clumps are colonies of candids organisms growing on the mucosa

neously within 10 days. The primary infection can occur in infancy and may be confused with teething. When young children are affected, they can become rapidly dehydrated and an adequate fluid intake is essential. As the virus often remains dormant in the tissues, secondary attacks can occur, either in the mouth or on the lips as **herpes labalis** or **cold sores**.

Ulceration can also be caused by trauma,

such as lip biting or by the sharp edge of a denture, however all innocent ulcers should heal within a month.

WHITE AND RED PATCHES

A number of conditions can present as white or red patches in the mouth. Some patches can be caused by simple friction from cheek biting, but others may be forms of chronic candidosis or pre-malignant conditions. Any white or red patch persisting for more than a few weeks should be investigated.

DRY MOUTH

Xerostomia, or dry mouth, is a common condition that can make eating or even speech difficult and can increase the risk of dental caries and periodontal disease. Although it can affect people of all ages, it appears to be more common in the elderly. However, recent research suggests that age, in itself, is not an important factor, but possibly the wide range of drugs that induce xerostomia as a side-effect and which many elderly people require. Specific causes of xerostomia include diabetes, a blocked salivary duct, chronic dehydration and more rarely, a salivary gland tumour or Sjogrens syndrome. A very severe form of xerostomia can follow from radiotherapy for tumours of the head or neck, as salivary glands are very sensitive to radiation. Rapidly progressive dental caries and periodontal disease can quickly follow and this condition requires the intensive application of preventive measures. Apart from treating any basic cause, artificial saliva can be used, but many sufferers find that the frequent sipping of iced water gives the best relief. Spicy foods should be avoided, however chewing sugar-free gum may provide relief.

There are some conditions arising elsewhere in the body that can have a visible effect within the mouth, such as pregnancy, anaemia and HIV infection (AIDS). These also need professional advice and help.

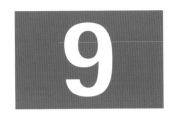
IN BRIEF
- Parents should supervise or assist with brushing until children can do it effectively, usually by the age of 7 years. Evidence Base C
- Low fluoride toothpastes provide only limited anti-caries benefit. Evidence Base A
- A child's normal fluid intake should ideally be plain water or milk. Evidence Base C

The scientific basis of oral health education. Part 9: Advice for children under five

R. S. Levine and C. R. Stillman-Lowe

TOOTHBRUSHING

Regular, twice daily, tooth brushing with a fluoride toothpaste can be introduced shortly after the appearance of the first teeth. However, in the Republic of Ireland, because of widespread water fluoridation, the advice is to begin brushing from 2 years of age, or use a non-fluoride toothpaste before 2 years. A small soft toothbrush should be used, with just a smear of toothpaste, increasing from the age of about 3 years, to a small pea-sized amount for children under 7 years. A gentle and systematic approach should be used with the aim of cleaning the outside, inside and biting surfaces of all teeth, including the back ones when they appear, usually between 1 and 2 years of age. Younger children are often quite happy to brush their own teeth, but lack the manual dexterity to do so efficiently. Parents should supervise or assist with brushing until the children can do it effectively, usually by the age of 7 years. However, some children need supervision beyond this age.

A fluoride toothpaste is recommended. Low fluoride toothpastes provide only limited anti-

caries benefit and unless the child and any siblings are caries-free and in good health, a regular family fluoride toothpaste should be used. However, care should be taken to ensure that younger children do not eat toothpaste directly from the tube or swallow excessive amounts from the brush.

DRINKS

Parents and carers of infants should be specifically warned against the practice of allowing prolonged drinking from a bottle, valve-type feeder or any other type of lidded feeder cup of any sugars-sweetened drink, including carbonated drinks, fruit-based juices, squash and natural fruit juice. The prolonged contact time between the sugar in the drink and the teeth is well recognised as a cause of rapidly progressing decay, usually of the upper front teeth, resulting in a condition, previously referred to as 'nursing bottle caries', but now termed 'early childhood caries' (Fig. 1). The risk from this practice is increased if the bottle is used to comfort the child, especially at bedtime or when in a cot or pushchair.

If sugars-sweetened drinks are given to younger children, they should be very well diluted, taken preferably at meal times only and drinking times should be kept short. An open cup or beaker should be used, never a bottle. Preferable alternatives are the lightly flavoured mineral waters, which state that they are suitable for infants. Parents and carers should be aware however that the sugar content of some flavoured bottled mineral waters can be as high as 10% and the precautions given above for sugars-sweetened drinks should be followed. A child's normal fluid intake should ideally be plain water or milk.

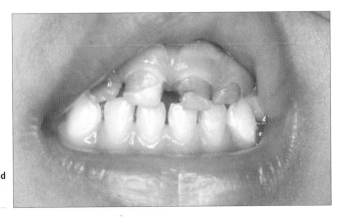

Fig. 1 Early childhood caries, better known as 'bottle caries'

Breast milk is the best form of nutrition for infants. When breastfeeding is not possible, cows' milk formulas are the preferred option. Infants and children should continue on hydrolysed protein infant formulas or soya infant formulas until they are 2 years old. Hydrolysed protein infant formulas are better nutritionally than those based on soya and infants with an allergy to cows' milk may also have an allergy to soya formula. However, mothers who have been advised by their GP or other health professional to feed their baby soya-based infant formulas, should continue to do so. Soya-based infant formulas contain sugars that can cause tooth decay, so it will be particularly important to be careful about caring for the baby's teeth once they start coming through.

IN BRIEF

- Everyone, including those with full dentures should have regular oral examinations. **Evidence Base C**
- Dentures should be removed and cleaned every night and should be replaced when damaged, ill-fitting or worn out. **Evidence Base C**

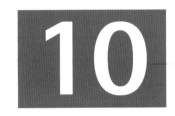

The scientific basis of oral health education.
Part 10: Advice for denture wearers and older people

R. S. Levine and C. R. Stillman-Lowe

While the number of denture wearers, especially full dentures, has steadily declined, it is estimated that by 2018, around 5% of the adult population will be edentulous and need full dentures (around two million people in the UK); a combination of natural teeth and dentures will still be as common as ever for the next 20 years. Demographic changes suggest an increasing proportion of these will be elderly and living either alone, possibly receiving community care, or in residential care or nursing care homes. The dental state of people in residential care is often poor, because help needed with oral hygiene may not be available. It is important that the wearers of full or partial dentures, and especially their carers, understand the need for special care if the health of their mouths and any remaining teeth are to be safeguarded.

DENTURE CLEANING

Routine care should include cleaning of the dentures after every meal and before going to bed. Ideally all dentures should be removed before sleeping to allow the soft tissues of the mouth to recover from the denture-bearing load and to remove the risk of injury or candida infection. Where this is not practical, they should be removed for at least 4 hours during the day. A small soft brush and a denture cleaning paste or liquid soap should be used to clean all denture surfaces before rinsing the denture and placing it in a hypochlorite based soaking solution of the *Steradent* type. Hypochlorite is bactericidal and fungicidal and helps to break down the organic matrix of adherent plaque that forms on the dentures, but can cause bleaching of denture plastic if dentures are soaked for long periods or in hot water. Hypochlorite is not suitable for metal-based dentures for which special soaking solu-

tions containing alkaline peroxide are available. After soaking, the dentures should be brushed and rinsed with water before being inserted. With all cleaning and soaking agents manufacturer's instructions should be carefully followed. It should be stressed that soaking alone will not clean dentures and thorough brushing before soaking is essential. Any natural teeth should be brushed twice daily with a fluoride toothpaste. The roof of the mouth, the gum ridges and tongue should be gently cleaned daily with a soft brush to remove any food particles and plaque.

Dentures, whether full or partial, do not last indefinitely. The ridges progressively change shape and the edges of the dentures can then begin to irritate the surrounding mucosa. This may cause the dentures to become loose or painful to wear. Even if they remain comfortable, the plastic teeth on the dentures wear down, causing the vertical height between nose and chin to be reduced and the lips to fall in. Often, dentures can be improved by relining the fitting surface, but sometimes older people do not take well to completely new dentures. However, if badly worn, broken or ill-fitting they should be replaced.

Because of these considerations, it is advised that denture wearers have their mouths and dentures examined at least every year. As the loss of a denture may cause great distress, especially for older people, dentists making dentures should be asked to include an embedded identification name.

ROOT CARIES

An increasing number of elderly people are retaining some or all of their natural teeth. Since many will have periodontal disease with gum recession, caries may develop on the exposed root surfaces. This is a common problem, made worse by reduced salivary flow and difficulty in maintaining good plaque control, especially round lower anterior teeth. Treating root caries can be difficult, especially in lower anterior teeth, but poor oral hygiene, possibly aggravated by ill-fitting partial dentures and periodontal disease, in an institutionalised elderly person in poor health, can result in a major clinical problem. For home care, careful and effective toothbrushing with a high concentration fluoride toothpaste is recommended, together with regular dental check-ups. If teeth are sensitive to hot and cold drinks, the use of a fluoride containing 'sensitive toothpaste' can give relief. However, if discomfort persists, then dental advice should be sought. The use of interdental brushes, especially for cleaning between the lower anterior teeth can be beneficial, but again dental advice should be sought.

Apart from problems related to teeth, gums and dentures, the elderly are more prone to dry mouth, possibly linked to their medication and candida infections of the mouth. It must be remembered that the majority of oral cancers occur in the over 60s. The proper dental care of the elderly, especially those in residential care homes, is increasingly a cause for concern. Oral health education for community care, residential and nursing care workers should be a part of their training and should be coordinated with local dental services.

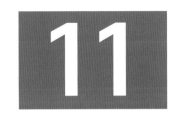

IN BRIEF
- There is no evidence that 6-monthly recalls are the optimum frequency. **Evidence Base C**
- Most people, irrespective of age and dental condition should have an oral examination about once a year. **Evidence Base C**
- The period between examinations should be determined on dental advice and reflect the individual risk of oral disease and medical, physical and social factors. **Evidence Base C**

The scientific basis of oral health education.
Part 11: Frequency of oral examinations

R. S. Levine and C. R. Stillman-Lowe

While it is accepted that oral examinations at appropriate intervals are of value in maintaining oral health, there is little evidence to support a specific interval or to quantify the benefit and no evidence that 6-monthly recalls are the optimum frequency.[1,2] There are now very many children and adults with little or no dental disease for whom frequent attendance is inappropriate. However, in some areas and among some social groups, the level of oral disease remains high while frequency of attendance is low.

The maintenance of periodontal health depends upon daily personal plaque control. Regular professional care may be required at intervals depending on the needs of the individual. With respect to decay, once a definite cavity is present, it cannot be remineralised, but the tooth can be restored and the importance of early detection and appropriate treatment makes dental attendance advisable. Other disorders can occur in the mouth which are unrelated to the presence of natural teeth and which may be life-threatening.

For all of these reasons, the period between oral examinations must be flexible and based on a professional assessment of the risk from oral disease. The period between oral examinations for everyone, irrespective of age or dental condition, should be about 1 year. This period can be extended for adults with no evidence of dental disease, who are in good general health and do not use tobacco and have low and infrequent sugar and alcohol consumption. Children may need to be seen more frequently, as may those who are at increased risk to oral disease because of smoking, medical, physical or social factors, or for whom dental treatment presents difficulties because of their medical or physical condition. Attendance will enable the health of the whole mouth to be monitored and appropriate dental health advice and early treatment to be provided when needed.

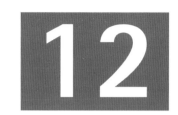

IN BRIEF
- Health education includes giving people personally relevant information about their health, which is based on a consensus of scientific evidence and opinion. **Evidence Base C**
- We have a responsibility to base health education programmes on the best available evidence of what works, and to evaluate interventions in order to strengthen the evidence-base and improve the quality of health education. **Evidence Base C**

The scientific basis of oral health education.
Part 12: Health education

R. S. Levine and C. R. Stillman-Lowe

WHAT IS HEALTH EDUCATION?

There are many definitions of health education, however one of the most useful is an adaptation of a definition from the World Health Organisation:

> 'Health education is the process by which people are given information to enable them to exercise a greater degree of control over their own health'.

The process of formulating and delivering health education messages includes a series of steps:

- The first step is to gain an understanding of the basic cause of the disease process under consideration. Taking dental caries as an example, the basic mechanism is the conversion of sugars in the diet into acid by the bacteria in plaque on the surfaces of the teeth.
- Next it is necessary to identify the essential causative factors. Some of these will be beyond individual personal control, such as genetically linked or environmental factors. However others may be under the control of the individual and amenable to change. In the case of caries, factors under personal control can include the effective use of fluoride toothpaste and the frequency of consumption of sugar-containing foods and drinks.
- The third stage is to agree scientifically based and socially acceptable messages for the public aimed at encouraging beneficial behavioural changes. For the prevention of dental caries one scientifically sound message would be that people should never consume sugars as part of their diet. However compliance with this message is quite unrealistic because sug-

ars are present in many foods and drinks, either naturally or artificially added. A more sensible message is to avoid sugars-sweetened food and drink between meals and at bedtime. This message can reduce the risk from tooth decay and is more likely to be accepted, though it may need to be modified further where individuals' eating patterns do not conform to traditional mealtimes, and there may be no regular fixed bedtime for children.

- The final, and possibly the most difficult stage of oral health education is that of communication. This process aims to ensure that key information is conveyed comprehensibly to the right target audience, in the right context, at the right time. In line with the World Health Organisation's Ottawa Charter, strategic aims for health promotion include traditional methods of health education, such as giving information and advice, thereby developing personal knowledge and skills. However, health promotion may also include other elements: building public policies that support health; creating supportive environments; strengthening community action; and re-orientating health services. These are beyond the scope of this book, but vital if health education initiatives are to be successful.

DOES HEALTH EDUCATION WORK?

One of the most debated issues in public health is the effectiveness of health education and promotion. Much public money is spent on a range of interventions, ranging from one-to-one advice in the GP surgery, to comprehensive healthy schools schemes, and mass media campaigns aimed for example at encouraging smoking cessation. The strength of the evidence-base for these interventions varies. A number of systematic reviews have examined studies in the dental field. Their findings were not always consistent, however the following conclusions were published in the report commissioned by Health Promotion Wales.[13]

- There is clear evidence that oral health education/promotion can be effective in bringing about changes in people's knowledge, and in improving people's oral health.
- It is unclear whether one-off oral health promotion initiatives are sufficient to improve individuals' oral health significantly for long periods.
- There is evidence that programmes using more innovative approaches than the Medical/ Behavioural model, have more potential for longer-term behaviour changes. They are more likely to be based on models of education and health behaviour which recognise the full variety of factors which influence a person's ability to comply with any messages given.
- Limited short-term behaviour changes are achievable using simple persuasive approaches. Greater or longer-term changes appear possible by using more tailored approaches that are based around active participation and addressing social, cultural and personal norms and values. The use of appropriate language and simple messages is important in avoiding confusion.
- Some studies show that health education which targets whole populations may increase inequalities in health.
- Preventive and comprehensive clinical approaches (including the appropriate use of fissure sealants) to oral health education can be effective in reducing the incidence of dental caries. However, this approach is intensive, and may not reach those in greatest need.
- Changing personal health behaviour appears to be more difficult for some groups than others; this may result in blaming the victim for not making the appropriate behaviour changes.
- Fluoride toothpaste is an important and effective method of delivering fluoride, although it will not reach the entire population. Evidence for the effectiveness of fluoride supplements, such as fluoride tablets, in home use and community schemes is at best equivocal and often shows them to be ineffective.

The Health Education Authority's review[14] concluded that:

- Oral health promotion, which includes the use of therapeutic agents incorporating fluoride (whether in the form of toothpaste, tablets, drops, gels or rinses) is effective in reducing the development of caries. These improvements are cumulative and increase over time. Daily brushing with fluoride toothpaste is easier to achieve than regular use of other fluoride supplements. There is no evidence that

oral health promotion per se affects caries rates, even if changes in behaviour are achieved, unless fluoride is being used.
- Clinical chairside advice and instruction aimed at improving oral hygiene have been shown to be effective.
- Oral health education on an individual level aimed at improving oral hygiene is capable of reducing plaque levels. However, there is strong evidence that changes achieved are short-term and are not sustained. Interventions are effective even when very simple direct instruction is used. Cognitive-behavioural techniques are not required in order to achieve changes in plaque levels.
- The evidence suggests that oral health promotion is effective in increasing knowledge levels, but there is no evidence that changes in knowledge are causally related to changes in behaviour. However, there would appear to be an ethical responsibility for scientific knowledge to be disseminated to the public, irrespective of what the population does with that knowledge.
- Attempts to control individuals' consumption of sweet foods and drinks are generally not satisfactorily evaluated. However, when such interventions are directed at individuals, they appear to be of limited value.

In an age when cost-benefit assumes growing importance in healthcare, the effectiveness of oral health education in terms of the reduction in disease and healthcare costs is clearly of great significance, when investing scarce resources. However, there is also an ethical obligation for health professionals possessing information that could reduce the prevalence of disease to inform the public accordingly, irrespective of whether a cost benefit can be proven to follow. The right of individuals to health education information was clearly defined by the Ottawa Charter in 1987.

Therefore three things are clear. Firstly, that more research is needed with the aims of improving the quality of health education delivered and evaluating the results of interventions, including their sustainability. The second is that although strong evidence for the effectiveness of health education and promotion is lacking in some areas, this does not remove from health professionals the responsibility to provide the public with all available information for the promotion of good health. Finally, in order to be effective, health education needs to be properly planned and organised, using the skills of the whole dental team, and the best quality and most appropriate resources.

WHICH TOPICS ARE INCLUDED IN THIS DOCUMENT?

Over the years, many requests had been received to include additional topics within *The Scientific Basis of Dental Health Education* document. To understand the problems involved in selecting topics for inclusion, it is helpful to consider possible topics under three headings:

Health education

Clinical chairside advice and instruction aimed at improving oral hygiene have been shown to be effective

- Topics where a substantial body of scientific evidence is available to support a useful health education statement. An example being the use of fluoride toothpaste.
- Topics where guidance for the public in the form of a health education message is required but where scientific evidence is lacking. Provided that there is a consensus of scientific opinion, a statement can be made, though this will be subject to change as new evidence and guidelines are published. An example being how often people should have a dental check-up.
- Topics that require guidance for the public but where there is neither a substantial body of scientific evidence nor a consensus of opinion amongst experts. If experts cannot agree then no statement can or should be given. An example is whether the teeth should be brushed before or after eating.

THE NATURE OF SCIENTIFIC EVIDENCE

Scientific evidence comes in many forms, but in the context of oral health it breaks down and into two main categories:

- *Laboratory-based studies.* These range from purely chemical or biological observations and experiments on the structure of teeth and the mouth, to experiments involving animals or small groups of human volunteers. Examples include the analysis of the changes that occur in teeth when they decay, and studies on the effect on bacteria in the mouth when human volunteers use different types of toothpaste.
- *Clinical studies.* These include observational studies where existing aspects of health are studied in large groups or populations without any form of intervention. These studies can include longitudinal ones where a group of subjects are followed over a period of time, cross-sectional studies and case-controlled studies where a comparison is made with a control group. An important type of clinical study is the interventional experiment. These studies are usually made up of at least two groups, one of which will be a control group who received no intervention and the other groups will follow some form of experimental regime. A good example is the clinical trial of a new toothpaste. In an ideal experiment subjects will be randomly allocated to a group and the research workers who make the observations will have no knowledge of the group to which any subject has been allocated. This type of experiment is called a randomised controlled trial (RCT) and has often been described as the gold standard for clinical research.

Good research studies are usually published in peer-reviewed scientific and clinical journals. These accept only those manuscripts which have been independently reviewed and refereed by experts in the field to ensure that the methods used and the conclusion that have been drawn are valid. A very useful overview of research in any particular field is often provided by a systematic review. This is usually written by leading experts who look at all the research that has been done, compare and contrast the results, possibly commenting on the quality of the research and draw appropriate conclusions. Finally, there is a method of comparing the results from a number of studies that have looked at the same issue, usually in the form of randomised controlled trials. Using a sophisticated statistical analysis the results from all of the trials are pooled together to arrive at one conclusion. This type of overall analysis of results is called a meta-analysis.

One very important point must be made about the result of any scientific research. When the conclusion of a study is that "there is no evidence to form a conclusion", it does not mean that the negative situation has been firmly established. It simply means that the experiment has not provided evidence for or against the relationship being studied. This is a point that is frequently misunderstood by those without a scientific background, who will reasonably assume that when a scientist says that there is no evidence for this or that, it means that it is not true. All the scientist is saying is that the experiment does not give any evidence to draw a conclusion. It is possible that next week or next year evidence will appear that does establish the case.

HEALTH EDUCATION AND EVIDENCE–BASED DENTISTRY

From the early 1970s there has been a growing interest in placing all aspects of clinical practice on an evidence-supported basis. One of the pioneers of this movement was Professor Archie Cochrane, who gave his name to an international collaborative network of groups with the aim of developing evidence based decision-making for clinical interventions. The Cochrane Network produces a series of systematic reviews of scientific evidence on a range of topics and some of these are used to support statements made in this document. A further extension of this movement is the appearance of a number of organisations and networks whose aim is to standardise and integrate the methods used for the development of guidelines for clinical practice. In the United Kingdom one of the most useful is that developed by the Scottish Inter-collegiate Guidelines Network (www.sign.ac.uk). One result of this work has been to establish a framework that enables those involved in producing clinical guidelines to formulate them on a common basis.

The concept of putting clinical practice on to an evidence basis has run in parallel with work to ensure that health education messages given to the public are based on sound scientific evidence. Nevertheless, an important difference

Topics included

Where there is either a substantial body of scientific evidence to support a useful health education statement, or a consensus of scientific opinion, then guidance for the public should be given

between these two areas is that while the evidence for clinical interventions ideally comes from high quality clinical studies such as a randomised controlled trials (RCT), the evidence to support dental health education messages often comes from laboratory based studies. Because of this difference a grading system for evidence relating to clinical interventions is not appropriate for grading the quality of evidence in relation to health education issues. A complex system for indicating levels of evidence has been developed by the Centre for Evidence-based Medicine in Oxford (CEM) and this scheme is undergoing constant refinement (www.ihs.ox.ac.uk/cebd). In this book, a simple scheme is introduced to give an indication of the volume and quality of evidence supporting key statements for dental health education and is

referred to as Evidence Bases. The equivalent nearest CEM levels are given in brackets.

- Level A: Statements supported by meta-analyses or systematic reviews (CEM levels 1 and 2)
- Level B: Statements supported by the majority of relevant research studies. (CEM level 3 and 4)
- Level C: Statements that cannot be supported by a substantial body of research evidence, but where there is a consensus of scientific and professional opinion to support the statement. There may nevertheless be dissenting views, as the issue may be the subject of continuing debate and ongoing research studies. (CEM level 5)

Where appropriate these grades are marked as Evidence Bases A, B and C, respectively.

Scientific Basis of Oral Health Education

List of key points

Chapter 1 Dental Caries

- Caries is caused by the action of sugars on the bacterial plaque covering the teeth. **Evidence Base   A**

- Caries occurs when demineralisation of the tooth surface exceeds remineralisation. **Evidence Base A**

- The risk of developing caries can be reduced by avoiding sugars between meals and at bedtime. **Evidence Base B**

- The risk of developing caries can be reduced by brushing with a fluoride toothpaste twice daily. **Evidence Base A**

- Never leave infants with sugars-sweetened drinks in feeding bottles or cups, especially at bedtime. **Evidence Base B**

- Caries occurs in all populations and age groups but is more common amongst children and disadvantaged groups. **Evidence Base A**

Chapter 2 Fluoride

- Twice daily brushing with fluoride toothpaste is an effective preventive measure, but requires compliance. **Evidence Base A**

- A small pea-sized amount of fluoride toothpaste should be used by young children (a small smear for babies) and brushing with fluoride toothpaste should be supervised. **Evidence Base C**

- Water fluoridation is safe and effective, but should be targeted at communities with higher caries levels where it is technically feasible. **Evidence Base A**

- Fluoride supplements, though shown to be effective in clinical trials, may not be as effective in practice for home use or in community schemes. **Evidence Base B**

Chapter 3 Diet and oral health

- The frequency and amount of consumption of sugars in drinks and foods are the most important risk factors for dental caries. **Evidence Base A**

- Sugars-sweetened snacks, cereals and drinks should be avoided between meals and especially at bedtime. **Evidence Base B**

- Naturally occurring sugars when consumed in fresh whole fruit, vegetables and cereal grains are not a risk factor for dental caries and these items are an essential part of a health balanced diet. **Evidence Base B**

Chapter 4 Periodontal disease

- The risk of developing periodontal disease can be reduced by careful and effective daily toothbrushing. **Evidence Base A**

- The risk of developing periodontal disease can be reduced by not smoking. **Evidence Base B**

Chapter 5 Plaque control and dental disease

- Twice daily brushing with a manual or powered toothbrush and a fluoride-containing toothpaste is the principal means of plaque control. **Evidence Base A**

- Other aids such as floss and interdental brushes can be highly effective but are best used following professional advice. **Evidence Base C**

Chapter 6 Erosion

- Limit the frequency of intake of acidic beverages. **Evidence Base B**

- Avoid brushing for one hour after an 'acidic' episode. **Evidence Base C**

Chapter 7 Oral cancer

- Smoking, other forms of tobacco use and frequent alcohol consumption are the main risk factor for oral cancer. **Evidence Base A**

- Oral ulceration present for more than three weeks requires immediate investigation. **Evidence Base C**

- Smokers who wish to give up should be given appropriate support to do so. **Evidence Base C**

Chapter 8 Other oral diseases

- Oral candidosis, when not associated with dentures, may be a sign of systemic disease causing immunosupression. **Evidence Base B**

- Dentures should be removed and cleaned every night and should be replaced when damage, ill-fitting or worn out. **Evidence Base C**

Chapter 9 Advice for children under 5

- Parents should supervise or assist with brushing until children can do it effectively, usually by the age of 7 years. **Evidence Base C**

- Low fluoride toothpastes provide only limited anti-caries benefit. **Evidence Base A**

- A child's normal fluid intake should ideally be plain water or milk. **Evidence Base C**

Chapter 10 Advice for denture wearers and the elderly

- Everyone, including those with full dentures should have regular oral examinations. **Evidence Base C**

- Denture should be removed and cleaned every night and should be replaced when damaged, ill-fitting or worn out. **Evidence Base C**

Chapter 11 Frequency of oral examinations

- Most people, irrespective of age and dental condition should have an oral examination about once a year. **Evidence Base C**

- The period between examinations should be determined on dental advice and reflect the risk of oral disease and medical, physical and social actors. **Evidence Base C**

- There is no evidence that 6-monthly recalls are the optimum frequency. **Evidence Base C**

Chapter 12 Health education

- Health education includes giving people personally relevant information about their health, which is based on a consensus of scientific evidence and opinion. **Evidence Base C**

- We have a responsibility to base health education programmes on the best available evidence of what works, and to evaluate interventions in order to strengthen the evidence-base and improve the quality of health education. **Evidence Base C**

Appendix 1 Smoking cessation and the dental team

- Smokers who wish to give up should be helped by the dental team to do so. **Evidence Base C**

Appendix 2 Guidelines for a healthy diet

- Dietary advice for patients given by the dental team should be consistent with general healthy eating guidelines. **Evidence Base C**

References

1. Pitts N B, Boyles J J, Nugent Z J. The dental caries experience of 5-year-old children in England and Wales. Surveys co-ordinated by the British Association for the Study of Community Dentistry in 2001/2002. *Community Dent Health* 2003; **20:** 49-54.

2. Pitts N B, Evans D J, Nugent Z J. The dental caries experience of 5-year-old children in the United Kingdom. Surveys co-ordinated by the British Association for the Study of Community Dentistry in1997/98. *Community Dent Health* 1999; **16:** 50-56.

3. Pine C, Burnside G, Craven R. Inequalities in dental health in the North-West of England. *Community Dent Health* 2003; **20:** 53-54.

4. Holt R D, Nunn J H, Rock W P, Page J. Fluoride Dietary Supplements and fluoride toothpaste for children. *Int J Paed dent* 1996; **6:** 139-142.

5. NHS Centre for Reviews and Dissemination. *Fluoridation of Drinking Water: a Systematic Review of its Efficacy and Safety* (Report No 18). York: University of York, 2000.

6. Department of Health. *Dietary Sugars and Human disease —Report of the Committee on Medical Aspects of Food Policy [COMA].* London: HMSO, 1989.

7. Maguire A, Rugg-Gunn A J. Xylitol and caries prevention — is it a magic bullet? *Br Dent J* 2003; **194:** 429-438.

8. Levine R S. Caries experience and bedtime consumption of sugar-sweetened foods and drinks — a survey of 600 children. *Community Dent Health* 2001; **18:** 228-231.

9. Heanue M, Deacon S A, Deery C, Robinson P G, Walmsley A D, Worthington H V, and Shaw W C. *Manual versus Powered Toothbrushing for Oral Health (Cochrane Review).* Cochrane Library, 2003. Issue 1. Oxford: Update Software.

10. O'Brian M. *Child Dental Health in the United Kingdom 1993.* Office of Population Census and Surveys. London: HMSO, 1994.

11. Cancer Research UK (2003), www.cancerresearchuk.org.

12. Davenport C F, Elley K M, Fry-Smith A, Taylor-Wheetman C L, Taylor R S. The effectiveness of routine dental checks; a systematic review of the evidence base. *Br Dent J* 2003; **195:** 87-98.

13. Sprod A J, Anderson A, Treasure E T. *Effective Oral Health Promotion: Literature review.* Technical Report 20. Cardiff: Health Promotion Wales, 1996.

14. Kay E J, Locker D. *Effectiveness of Oral Health Promotion: a Review.* London: Health Education Authority, 1997.

Further reading

(in alphabetical order)

Blinkhorn A. Oral health education. *In* Seward M H and Rothwell P S (eds) *Oral Health Promotion with Teamwork.* Sheffield: Teamwork Publications,1997.

Clarkson J, Harrison J E, Ismail A I, Needleman I, Worthington H. *Evidence Based Dentistry for Effective Practice.* London: Martin Dunitz, 2003.

The Dairy Council. *Topical Update: Diet and Dental Health.* London: The Dairy Council, 2001.

Davies R M, Davies G M, Ellwood R P. Prevention. Part 4: Toothbrushing: what advice should be given to patients? *Br Dent J* 2003; **195:** 135-141.

Daly B, Watt R G, Batchelor P and Treasure E T. *Essential Dental Public Health.* Oxford: OUP, 2002.

Department of Health. *Dietary sugars and human disease.* Report of the Committee on Medical Aspects of Food Policy [COMA]. London: HMSO, 1989.

Department of Health. *Weaning and The Weaning Diet.* Report of the Working Group on the Weaning Diet of the Committee on Medical Aspects of Food Policy [COMA]. London; HMSO, 1994.

Department of Health (1997). *Statement on Sugar, formulated by COMA.* Published in Food Safety Information Bulletin, and available at www.doh.gov.uk/coma/state.htm

Department of Health. Modernising NHS Dentistry. *In Implementing the NHS Plan.* London: HMSO, 2000.

Fejerskov O, Nyvad B, Kidd E A M. Clinical and histological manifestations of dental caries. *In* Fejerskov O and Kidd E A M (eds) *Dental caries the disease and its clinical management.* pp71-98. Oxford: Blackwell Munksgaard, 2003.

Health Development Agency. *Standard for Training in Smoking Cessation treatments.* London: Health Development Agency, 2003.

Health Education Authority. *Sugars in the diet.* London: Health Education Authority, 1999.

Health Technology and Assessment NHS R & D HTA Programme report on *The clinical effectiveness and cost-effectiveness of routine dental checks: a systematic review and economic evaluation,* by Davenport C, Elley K, Salas C, Taylor-Weetman C L, Fry-Smith A, Bryan S and Taylor R. Executive Summary, Health Technology Assessment 2003; Vol 7: No 7.

Holbrook W P, Arnadottir I B. Prevention. Part 3: Prevention of tooth wear. *Br Dent J* 2003; **195:** 75-81.

Jenkins W M M, Heasman P A The prevention and control of periodontal disease. *In* Murray J J, Nunn J H, Steele J G (eds.) *The Prevention of Oral Disease.* 4th edn, pp. 123-144. Oxford: Oxford Medical Publications, 2003.

Kent G, Croucher R. *Achieving Oral Health: the social context of dental care.* Oxford: Wright, 1998.

Marinho V C, Higgins J P, Sheiham A, Logan S. Fluoride toothpastes for preventing dental caries in children and adolescents (Cochrane Review). *Cochrane Database Syst Rev* 2003: CD002278.

Moynihan P J. Dietary advice in dental practice. *Br Dent J* 2002; **193:** 563-568.

Moynihan P J. Diet and Dental Caries. *In* Murray J J Nunn J H and Steele J G (eds.) *The Prevention of Oral Disease.* 4th edn, pp. 10-34. Oxford: Oxford Medical Publications, 2003.

Murray J J, Rugg-Gunn A J, Jenkins, G N. *Fluorides in Caries Prevention.* 3rd edn. Oxford: Butterworth-Heinemann, 1991.

Nuttal N, Steele J G, Nunn J, Pine C, Treasure E, Bradnock G, Morris J, Kelly M, Pitts N B, White D. *A Guide to the UK Adult Dental Health Survey 1998.* London: BDJ Books, 2001.

Palmer R T M, Floyd, P D. Periodontology: a clinical approach. 3: Non-surgical treatment and maintenance. *Br Dent J* 1995; 178: 263-268.

Pine C (ed). *Community Oral Health.* Oxford: Wright, 1997.

Royal College of Physicians of London. *Fluoride, Teeth and Health.* Tunbridge Wells: Pitman Medical, 1976.

Rugg-Gunn A J, Nunn J. *Nutrition, Diet and Oral Health.* Oxford: Oxford University Press, 1999.

Sheiham A. Dietary effects on dental diseases. *Public Health Nutrition* 2001; **4:** 569-591.

Sutcliffe P. Oral cleanliness and dental caries. *In* Murray J. J. (ed.) *The Prevention of Dental Disease.* 3rd edn, pp68-77. Oxford: Oxford Medical Publications, 1996.

Steele J, Walls A. Prevention in the ageing population. *In* Murray J J Nunn J H, Steele J G (eds.) *The Prevention of Oral Disease.* 4th edn, pp. 190-207. Oxford: Oxford Medical Publications, 2003.

ten Cate J M, Imfeld T (eds.) Etiology, mechanism and implications of dental erosion. *Eur J Oral Sci* 1996; **104:** (2, Pt. 2).

Watt R G, Daly B. *Prevention. Part 1: Smoking cessation advice within the general dental practice. Br Dent J* 2003; **194:** 665-668.

Watt R G , McGlone P. Prevention. Part 2: Dietary advice in the dental surgery. *Br Dent J* 2003; **195:** 27-31.

West R, McNeill A, Raw M. Smoking cessation guidelines for health professionals: an update. *Thorax* 2000; **55:** 987-999.

WHO. *Diet in the Prevention of Chronic Disease.* Technical Report Series 916. Geneva: WHO, 2003.

Scientific Basis of Oral Health Education

Appendices

Appendix 1 Smoking cessation and the dental team

Smoking remains the greatest preventable cause of disease and early death in England, and one of the greatest causes of the health divide between rich and poor. It is an addictive behaviour with strong social associations and is very difficult to stop. Overall, the government aims to persuade smokers to give up, to aid them in doing so, and to persuade non-smokers, particularly children, not to start. Smoking cessation interventions delivered through the NHS are an extremely cost effective way of preserving life and reducing ill health. GPs and practice nurses should receive training to enable them to deliver opportunistic advice to smokers. Smokers contacting the NHS should be asked about smoking and have the NHS smoking cessation services brought to their attention. Those who want to stop should be offered a package of both pharmaceutical aids and behavioural support to meet their particular needs and circumstances. Smokers should have access to a specialist smoking cessation service, and where this is not a desirable option, then other means of support should be discussed (such as telephone and self-help). The National Institute of Clinical Excellence (NICE) has recommend-ed the use of NRT (nicotine replacement therapy) or bupropion (Zyban) for smokers who wish to quit.

Although evidence is currently lacking for most professional groups, other primary healthcare team professionals should routinely:

- Ask their patients about smoking
- Advise smokers to stop
- Recommend sources of support where appropriate.

A protocol for the dental team to follow is given below (Fig. 1). It has been estimated that between 63,000 and 190,000 smokers would stop smoking in a year if all dentists routinely offered smoking cessation advice. Dental professionals offering smoking cessation treatments to patients, including brief interventions, should receive training to equip them with the knowledge and skills necessary to do so effectively.

Key Point:
- Smokers who wish to give up should be helped by the dental team to do so. **Evidence Base C**

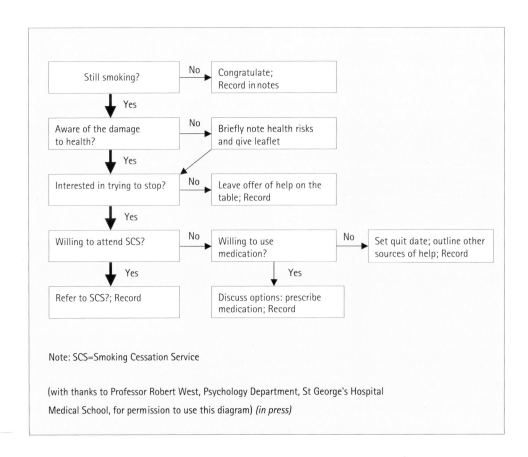

Note: SCS=Smoking Cessation Service

(with thanks to Professor Robert West, Psychology Department, St George's Hospital Medical School, for permission to use this diagram) *(in press)*

Fig. 1 Flowchart for brief advice to smokers

Appendix 2 Guidelines for a healthy diet

The Food Standards Agency (www.food.gov.uk) states that the key to a healthy diet is to eat a variety of foods, which for most people means eating:

- More fruit and vegetables
- More bread, cereals, and potatoes
- Less fat, sugar and salt.

  In more detail, adults should:

- Aim to make up a third of their diet from bread and cereals, choosing wholegrain, wholemeal, brown or 'high fibre' varieties whenever possible.
- Eat at least five portions of fruit and vegetables every day, including fresh, frozen, tinned, dried or juiced. Fruit and vegetables should make up about a third of the food eaten each day.
- Eat a moderate amount of meat, fish and alternatives such as pulses, eggs, nuts and beans, choosing lower fat versions when possible. At least two portions of fish per week should be eaten, one of which should be oily fish.
- Consume less fatty and sugary foods and drinks such as margarine, butter, cream, chocolate and biscuits, and soft drinks, sweets, jam, cakes and ice cream.
- Have milk, cheese, yoghurt, fromage frais and other dairy products in moderate amounts, choosing lower fat versions whenever possible
- Eat less salty foods. Most adults are eating too much (on average 9g of salt per day – two teaspoonfuls – which should be reduced to less than 6g). Most (about 75%) of the salt in our diets comes from processed foods.
- Drink alcohol only in moderation. Women can drink up to 2–3 units per day, and men up to 3–4 units per day, without significant risk to their health. Binge drinking should be avoided. Light to moderate drinking of one to two units of alcohol a day has a beneficial protective effect against coronary heart disease for men over 40 and women who have gone through the menopause.

Key Point:
Dietary advice for patients given by the dental team should be consistent with general healthy eating guidelines. Evidence Base C

Appendix 3 Eruption dates of teeth

Deciduous teeth (months)

Incisors	Canines	1st Molars	2nd Molars
6-8	12–20	12–16	20–30

Permanent teeth (years)

	Lower	Upper
1st Incisor	6–7	7–8
2nd Incisor	7–8	8–9
Canine	9–10	11–12
1st Premolar	9–12	9–12
2nd Premolar	10–12	10–12
1st Molar	6–7	6–7
2nd Molar	10–12	11–13
3rd Molar	17–21	17–21

Appendix 4 First aid for traumatised incisor teeth

It is estimated that about 10% of the population have at least one permanent incisor tooth affected by trauma by the age of 15 years and that many remain untreated. These injuries range from the minor, where the teeth can be restored easily by a dentist, to cases when one or more whole teeth are knocked out.

The following advice can be given:

- Professionally made mouthguards should be worn during sporting activities.
- If teeth are fractured, seek immediate dental help and avoid hot or cold liquids and foods.
- If a permanent tooth is knocked out and found, immediate re-implantation can be attempted. The tooth should be held by the crown and contact with the root should be avoided. Any contamination should be removed by rinsing with milk or tap water, but no attempt to clean or disinfect the tooth should be made. The tooth should be supported by biting on a clean folded handkerchief or tissue until seen by a dentist. Re-implantation should not be attempted for deciduous teeth, or if there is any doubt concerning the medical history of the individual.
- If re-implantation is not attempted, the tooth should be placed in a container of saliva or cold milk and taken to a dentist.
- Bleeding should be controlled by biting on a clean handkerchief or tissue for 20 minutes.
- Delay in seeking advice can result in the loss of teeth, which could be saved, or where teeth are knocked out, the movement of adjacent teeth could make the provision of false teeth more difficult.

Appendix 5 Useful evidence-based dentistry websites

- Centre for Evidence-based Dentistry **www.ihs.ox.ac.uk/cebd**

- Cochrane Oral Health Group **www.cochrane.org**

- NHS Centre for Reviews and Dissemination, University of York **www.nhscrd.york.ac.uk**

- National Co-ordinating Centre for Health Technology Assessment, Health Technology Assessment Programme **www.ncchta.org**

- National Electronic Library for Health – specialist library – Oral Health (dentistry) **www.nelh.nhs.uk/oralhealth/dental**

- National Institute for Clinical Excellence (NICE) **www.nice.org.uk**

- Royal College of Surgeons, Faculty of Dental Surgery **www.rcseng.ac.uk/dental/fds/clinical_guidelines/**

- Scottish Intercollegiate Guidelines Network (SIGN) **www.sign.ac.uk**

Appendix 7 List of expert advisers

Prof. A S Blinkhorn	Department of Child Dental Health, University of Manchester
Dr V Clerehugh	Department of Periodontology, University of Leeds
Dr S Creanor	Department of Adult Dental Health, University of Glasgow
Prof. E A M Kidd	GKT Dental Institute, University of London.
Prof. M A Lennon	Department of Oral Health and Development, University of Liverpool
Dr P J Moynihan	Department of Oral Biology and Child Dental Health, University of Newcastle upon Tyne
Prof. D O'Mullane	Department of Oral Health and Development, University of Cork
Prof. A Sheiham	University College Medical School, University of London
Prof. P M Speight	Department of Oral Pathology, University of Sheffield
Prof. E T Treasure	Dental Public Health Unit, University of Cardiff
Dr R G Watts	University College Medical School, University of London

Appendix 6 List of bodies and individuals responding to the consultation

The following bodies and individuals provided comments on this book at the draft stage. Their valuable contributions, representing a broad spectrum of expertise, were gratefully received.

The British Association for the Study of Community Dentistry
The British Association of Dental Nurses
The British Dental Association
The British Dental Health Foundation
The British Dental Hygienists' Association
The Conference of Postgraduate Dental Deans and Directors
The Department of Health
The Faculty of General Dental Practitioners of the Royal College of Surgeons
The Food Standards Agency
The General Dental Council
The National Association of Dentists in Health Authorities and Trusts
The National Oral Health Promotion Group

Ann Davies
Sabrina Fuller
Karen Gonzales
Charlotte Jeavons
Judi McGaffin
Sarah Murray
Mary O'Farrell
Dr T K Ong
Patti Speedy

Index